W9-BDY-474

Macular Degeneration

A Patient's Guide to Treatment

David S. Boyer, M.D.
Homayoun Tabandeh, M.D.

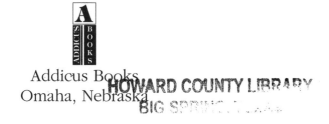

Addicus Books
Omaha, Nebraska

HOWARD COUNTY LIBRARY
BIG SPRING, TEXAS

An Addicus Nonfiction Book

Copyright 2012 by David S. Boyer, M.D., and Homayoun Tabandeh, M.D. All rights reserved. No part of this publication may be reproduced, stored in a retrieval system, or transmitted in any form or by any means, electronic, mechanical, photocopied, recorded, or otherwise, without the prior written permission of the publisher. For information, write Addicus Books, Inc., P.O. Box 45327, Omaha, Nebraska 68145.

ISBN 978-1-936374-32-8
Design by Jack Kusler
Illustrations by Jack Kusler

This book is not intended to be a substitute for a physician, nor do the authors intend to give advice contrary to that of an attending physician.

Library of Congress Cataloging-in-Publication Data

Boyer, David, 1947-
Macular degeneration : a patient's guide to treatment /
David Boyer, Homayoun Tabandeh.
    p. cm.
Includes bibliographical references and index.
ISBN 978-1-936374-32-8 (alk. paper)
1. Retinal degeneration. 2. Retinal degeneration—Treatment.
3. Self-care, Health. I. Tabandeh, Homayoun. II. Title.
RE661.D3B69 2011
617.7'35—dc23
                                                    2011041816

Addicus Books, Inc.
P.O. Box 45327
Omaha, Nebraska 68145
www.AddicusBooks.com

Printed in the United States of America
10 9 8 7 6 5 4 3 2 1

To the many people who are affected by macular degeneration; to our patients, who entrusted their care to us and inspired us to write this book; and to our families, whose support made this project possible.

Contents

Acknowledgments vii

Introduction ix

1   Macular Degeneration: An Overview 1

2   Symptoms and Signs of Macular Degeneration . 23

3   Getting a Diagnosis 32

4   Treatments for Macular Degeneration 54

5   Reducing the Risk of
    Macular Degeneration Progression 72

6   Living with Macular Degeneration 79

Appendix 97

Resources 99

Glossary 103

Index 113

About the Authors 123

Acknowledgments

We are grateful to our patients, who, through sharing their experiences, have educated us to see beyond the clinical manifestations of macular degeneration. Their endeavors have helped us understand macular degeneration as a condition not just affecting the macula, but the individual. We hope this book will help those with macular degeneration with the many challenges that they face daily.

We would like to express our gratitude to the many colleagues who graciously entrusted us with their patients' care. We would like to thank Adam Smucker and all the employees at the Retina-Vitreous Associates Medical Group, whose hard work and dedication to patient care have helped our patients and us tremendously. Our thanks also go to Frances Sharpe, Rod Colvin, Jack Kusler, and Addicus Books for their expert support of this project.

Introduction

Macular degeneration is a leading cause of vision loss in people over the age of fifty. According to the Macular Degeneration Foundation, more than two hundred thousand people are diagnosed with macular degeneration every year in the United States. As retina specialists, we diagnose and treat people with macular degeneration on a daily basis. The number of individuals who are suffering from the vision problems associated with macular degeneration is rising, keeping pace with our aging population. As the number of people entering their Golden Years continues to grow, an even greater number of people will be facing this condition.

With macular degeneration becoming more commonplace, many people want to understand more about it. If you or a loved one has been diagnosed with macular degeneration, you will naturally have many questions, both about the disease itself and the hurdles you or your loved one may face in the future. In this book, we attempt to provide a comprehensive, yet concise and easy-to-read, overview of macular degeneration, its causes, its symptoms, and the current treatments. Although at present there is no cure for macular degeneration, advances in treatment are offering more hope than ever before. Today, doctors have ways to delay the progression of the disease, to reduce the damage it can cause, to protect or even improve vision, and to help people adapt to the challenges it presents.

This book provides you and your family with the information you need to understand the basics of macular degeneration. It will help you understand what is involved in getting a diagnosis, taking an active role in your treatment, reducing your risk factors for progression of the disease, and living with macular degeneration.

1   Macular Degeneration: An Overview

Macular degeneration is a condition that causes deterioration of the *macula,* a small section of the retina that is responsible for sharp, central vision. With this condition, central vision deteriorates. It is estimated that as many as 11 million people in the United States have some form of *macular degeneration,* which is also known as *age-related macular degeneration (AMD).* In the United States, macular degeneration is the most common cause of vision loss in people over age fifty. In people under age fifty, there is only a 2 percent chance of developing macular degeneration. But by the time a person reaches age seventy-five, that risk jumps to nearly 30 percent. With our aging population, the number of people with macular degeneration is expected to skyrocket in the coming decades. In fact, it is estimated that by 2050, up to 22 million people will suffer from macular degeneration.

How the Human Eye Works

To fully understand macular degeneration and how it develops, it is a good idea to first look at how the human eye works. One of the easiest ways to understand the inner workings of the eye is to think of it as a camera.

The *cornea* is the clear, dome-shaped front part of the eye that works with the *lens* of the eye to act as the camera's lens, or focusing system. The *retina,* a very thin layer of light-sensitive tissue lining the inside of the back of the eye, is the film. In order to provide clear, distortion-free pictures, the film in a camera— or in this case, the retina—must be completely flat. If the film—or the retina—is damaged in any way or has any irregularities, the images will not be crystal clear; there may be distortion, blurring, or other problems.

Parts of the retina and surrounding tissues include the following:

- *Macula:* The macula is the center part of the retina and is critical for central vision, which is used to perform activities that require seeing fine detail, such as reading, watching television, driving, and recognizing faces at a distance. The macula is also what allows us to see our world in color.
- *Fovea:* At the center of the macula is a tiny dimple known as the fovea. The most sensitive portion of the macula, the fovea is responsible for our sharpest vision.
- *Choroid:* In a healthy eye, the retina lies over a flat carpet of blood vessels called the choroid. The choroid supplies the retina with nourishment.
- *Retinal pigment epithelium:* A single layer of very specialized cells called the retinal pigment epithelium (RPE) buffers the retina from the choroid.

- *Bruch's membrane:* Lying between the RPE and the choroid is a thin, semipermeable membrane called Bruch's membrane, which serves as an additional protective buffer between the retina and the choroid.

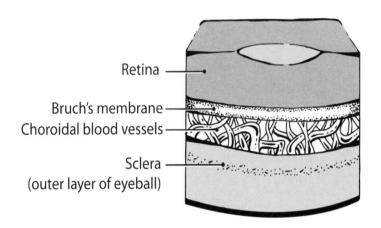

Normal Retina: Oxygen, micronutrients, and cellular waste flow through Bruch's membrane.

Nutrients traveling from the choroid blood vessels to the retina must pass through Bruch's membrane and then through the retinal pigment epithelium. On the other hand, waste products generated by the retina must pass through the retinal pigment epithelium and then through Bruch's membrane in order to be transported away by the blood vessels in the choroid. This inflow of nutrients and outflow of waste products, or debris, occurs twenty-four hours a day to keep the retina healthy.

How Macular Degeneration Develops

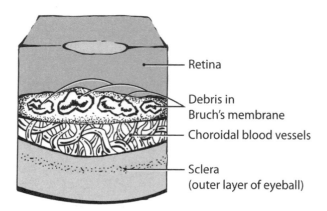

Retina

Debris in Bruch's membrane

Choroidal blood vessels

Sclera (outer layer of eyeball)

Dry Macular Degeneration: Debris in Bruch's membrane impedes the flow of oxygen, micronutrients, and cellular waste.

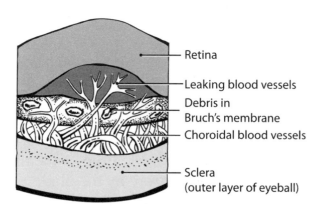

Retina

Leaking blood vessels

Debris in Bruch's membrane

Choroidal blood vessels

Sclera (outer layer of eyeball)

Wet Macular Degeneration: Abnormal, fragile blood vessels that grow under the retina leak blood and other fluids. This damages the overlying retina and affects vision.

As the Eye Ages

With aging, Bruch's membrane tends to thicken, disturbing the delicate balance of nutrients and debris. The flow of nutrients slows, and debris may begin to accumulate within the fibers of Bruch's membrane. The debris can form into small, yellow mounds called *drusen*. It is believed that all people will accumulate some debris in Bruch's membrane during their lifetime, but only some will develop drusen. The thickening of Bruch's membrane and the accumulation of drusen contribute to the development of macular degeneration. Other conditions associated with the development of the disease include degenerative changes in the retinal pigment epithelium, in the blood vessels in the choroid, and in the light-sensitive *photoreceptors* in the retina. Photoreceptors are retinal cells which detect light and enable us to see.

Types of Macular Degeneration

There are two basic types of macular degeneration: *dry macular degeneration* and *wet macular degeneration*. Dry macular degeneration is the most common form, affecting up to 90 percent of people with macular degeneration. There are three stages of dry macular degeneration: early, intermediate, and advanced. Dry macular degeneration can develop into wet macular degeneration, which is considered to be the advanced form of the disease. However, only about 10 percent of patients with mild dry macular degeneration will develop the wet form of the disease. Patients with severe, or high-risk, dry macular degeneration have a 30 to 50 percent chance of developing wet macular degeneration within five years of their initial diagnosis.

Dry Macular Degeneration

Dry macular degeneration is a chronic condition that affects the macula. It can lead to vision problems, such as blurring or blank spots, in the central field of vision.

Dry macular degeneration is characterized by a number of changes in the eye. One of the most common early changes is the accumulation of drusen, or small mounds of debris, in the membrane below the retina, Bruch's membrane. Other changes include the gradual breakdown of the tissues below the retina and the light-sensitive cells in the retina. Dry macular degeneration may also cause the degeneration of the small blood vessels in the choroid below the retina. In some cases, these changes are mild and may not produce any noticeable symptoms. In other cases, the changes are more pronounced and may lead to problems with vision.

In more-severe cases of dry macular degeneration, the loss of tissues and blood vessels may occur around the macula in a patchy pattern. This is called *geographic atrophy* and represents a more advanced form of dry macular degeneration. With this form, central vision problems may be mild, moderate, or severe, but tend to evolve gradually.

Wet Macular Degeneration

Wet macular degeneration occurs when abnormal blood vessels grow under the retina. These blood vessels originate from the small blood vessels in

Anatomy of the Eye

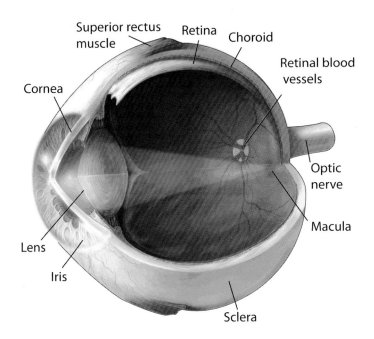

Retina and Macula

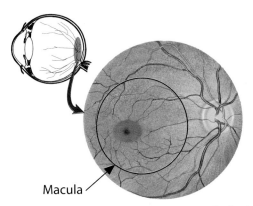

A close-up view of the retina and macula, which sit at the back of the eye, as shown in the small black and white illustration on the left.

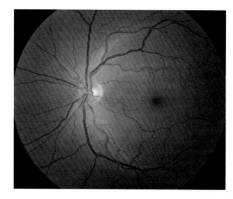

A normal retina with healthy macula, blood vessels, and optic nerve.

With dry macular degeneration, small mounds of debris (drusen)—the yellow spots toward the center of the eye—affect vision.

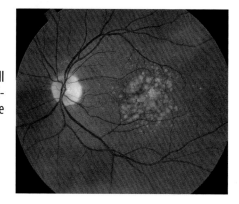

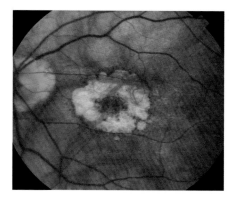

Macular geographic atrophy—the yellow patch in the center of the eye—is a severe form of dry macular degeneration. It's caused by deterioration of tissues and blood vessels.

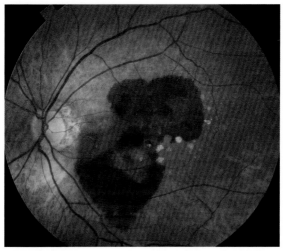

A severe case of wet macular degeneration with bleeding under the macula.

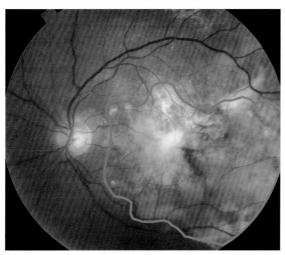

In severe wet macular degeneration, bleeding vessels may cause scarring, known as disciform scarring, which can profoundly affect central vision. The area outlined in blue shows the scarring.

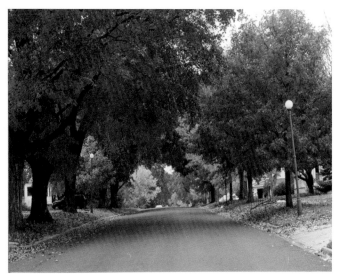

This photo represents normal vision. The image is clear and without obstruction.

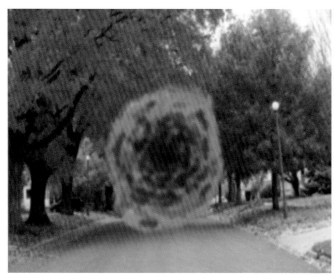

The blotch in this photo represents the type of central vision loss that is common with macular degeneration.

the choroid under the retina. This process is called *choroidal neovascularization (CNV)*. Unlike healthy blood vessels, these abnormal blood vessels are fragile, causing them to leak blood or other fluids under the retina. Leakage builds up under the retina, damaging it and causing the macula to bulge or lift away from the retina, resulting in an uneven surface. Remember, like the film in a camera, the retina must be flat in order to produce clear images. When it takes on an irregular shape, images become distorted and blurred. In addition, when blood or other fluids build up under the retina, the retina's light-detecting photoreceptors become damaged and cannot function normally.

With wet macular degeneration, these changes can occur very suddenly and may result in dramatic visual impairment. Although wet macular degeneration affects only about 10 percent of all people with macular degeneration, it accounts for more than two-thirds of significant vision loss among people with macular degeneration.

In wet macular degeneration, the choroidal neovascularization, or CNV, is subclassified into three types: classic, occult, or a mix of the two.

Classic

Classic wet macular degeneration occurs when abnormal blood vessels (resulting from CNV) rapidly leak blood or other fluids into the tissues under the retina, potentially causing sudden and significant problems with central vision.

Occult

Occult wet macular degeneration is associated with less-pronounced leakage of blood or other fluids into the tissues under the retina. This has a less dramatic impact on the shape of the macula and produces less-severe visual impairment initially. Although vision problems also occur at a slower pace with this type, occult wet macular degeneration can eventually cause major macular bleeding and loss of central vision.

Combination of Classic and Occult

The third type of wet macular degeneration is basically a combination of the classic and the occult types. With this combination type, there may be rapid leakage in some parts of the eye and less-pronounced leakage in other areas of the eye.

Approximately 90 percent of all cases of wet macular degeneration are predominantly occult or a combination of classic and occult. With the new treatments for wet macular degeneration, the distinction between the classic and the occult forms of the condition has become less important, as both types respond well to the treatments.

Retinal Pigment Epithelial Detachment

Retinal pigment epithelial detachment (PED) is a condition in which fluid builds up behind the thin layer of tissues under the retina, causing a small "blister" to develop under the macula. In wet macular degeneration, this condition occurs because of the growth of abnormal blood vessels under the retinal pigment epithelium. It is thought that people who have this condition may have a slower response to treatment for wet macular degeneration. Apart from wet macular degeneration, many other retina and choroid conditions can cause retinal pigment epithelial detachment.

Macular Scarring

In wet macular degeneration, macular scarring occurs as a result of leakage of blood or other fluids under the macula. The scarring permanently damages the overlying retina and causes reduced vision. The aim of treatment for wet macular degeneration is to stabilize the fragile abnormal blood vessels so that macular scarring is prevented or minimized. The smaller the area of scarring, the better the final vision.

Severe macular scarring, also called *disciform scarring*, is the end stage of wet macular degeneration. By this stage, central vision may be severely affected, depending on the location of the scar tissue relative to the fovea (the center of the macula). Currently, there are no effective treatments for macular scarring.

Other Effects of Wet Macular Degeneration
Vitreous Hemorrhage

An uncommon effect of wet macular degeneration is bleeding that invades the *vitreous*, the clear, jellylike substance that fills the inside of the eye. This type of bleeding is called a *vitreous hemorrhage*, and it can cause sudden impairment of both central vision and peripheral vision, which is the ability to see objects and movement outside the direct line of vision. Fortunately, with treatment, peripheral vision may be restored. Without treatment, vision loss can be permanent.

Visual Hallucinations

Visual hallucinations may occur in individuals who have moderate to severe vision loss in both eyes. These hallucinations may be simple patterns, colors, or lights, or may include formed and vivid visual images. The condition of visual hallucinations associated with poor vision is called *Charles Bonnet syndrome.* The syndrome is named after the Swiss naturalist and philosopher Charles Bonnet, who described the condition in the eighteenth century. Bonnet first documented the condition in his eighty-nine-year-old grandfather, who was blind from cataracts in both eyes but perceived images of men, women, birds, carriages, buildings, and tapestries.

Although Charles Bonnet syndrome occurs commonly in people with wet macular degeneration and poor vision, it is underdiagnosed. Characteristics of the syndrome include hallucinations in which the characters or objects are smaller than normal and often fit into the person's surroundings. The hallucinations are only visual and do not involve any other senses. The hallucinations may last only a few seconds or continue for hours. They occur more frequently in dim or dark lighting, such as in the evening. People who have this condition understand that the hallucinations are not real.

It is estimated that 10 to 40 percent of adults over age sixty-five with significant vision loss experience Charles Bonnet syndrome. However, many affected individuals may be reluctant to report the symptoms to their family members or doctors, out of fear that they will be labeled insane.

There is no treatment of proven effectiveness for this condition. It usually disappears within two years, although periodic relapses may occur. For those experiencing visual hallucinations, awareness that this is a known and common phenomenon, and not a mental illness, can alleviate distress and improve their ability to cope with the hallucinations. There are also a few activities that may help stop hallucinations, such as increasing the surrounding lighting or interrupting vision for a short time by closing the eyes or blinking. In some severe cases, medications such as selective serotonin reuptake inhibitors may be helpful.

Risk Factors for Macular Degeneration

It is not known exactly why some people develop macular degeneration and others do not, but it is thought that certain physical traits and lifestyle factors make some individuals more vulnerable to the disease. These are called risk factors. The more risk factors you have, the greater your chance of developing this condition. Many risk factors also tend to speed up the progression of macular degeneration. That's why it's important to understand and control the risk factors for this disease. By doing so, you can reduce your risk of developing macular degeneration or of the disease progressing.

Age

Age is the greatest risk factor for macular degeneration. It is uncommon to develop macular degeneration prior to age fifty. After that age, however, the risk begins to increase and continues to rise as your age advances. By the time an individual reaches age seventy-five, he or she has a 30 percent chance of developing macular degeneration. Because age is the most significant risk factor, it is important that all individuals over age fifty self-test their eyes on a regular basis for signs of macular degeneration and visit an eye care professional at least once a year.

Ethnicity

Macular degeneration occurs in all races but is more common in Caucasians than in nonwhites. However, scientists are now reporting that Asians may develop macular degeneration at nearly the same rate as Caucasians, who are more likely than African-Americans to experience vision loss from macular degeneration.

Gender

Women appear to be more likely to develop macular degeneration than men and, because they tend to live longer than men, are also more apt to experience vision loss. This does not mean that men do not need to be concerned about macular degeneration. Regardless of gender, everyone over age fifty should regularly self-test for signs of macular degeneration.

Family History

Mounting evidence suggests that a person's genes may play a role in the risk for this eye condition. A family history of macular degeneration is present in nearly three out of four cases of macular degeneration, according to research. Scientists believe that several genes may be associated with increased risk.

If any of your immediate family members has macular degeneration, your chance of developing it is two to three times greater than for people whose immediate family members do not have the disease. If one (or more) of your first-degree relatives has advanced macular degeneration, you have a 50 percent chance of developing it, as well.

Smoking

Current smokers are at greater risk for the disease and are more likely to develop advanced macular degeneration than nonsmokers. Quitting smoking is one of the best measures an individual can take to decrease the risk for this vision-threatening condition. Within the first year of quitting smoking, the chance of developing macular degeneration is reduced. The longer a person remains smoke-free, the lower the risk.

Cardiovascular Factors

A history of heart disease, stroke, or hardening of the arteries (arteriosclerosis) makes a person more vulnerable to macular degeneration. This association also goes the other way—people who have macular degeneration are more likely to have heart disease.

A growing body of scientific evidence shows that having risk factors for cardiovascular disease— even though cardiovascular disease itself is not present—also puts a person at higher risk for macular degeneration. In particular, researchers have found an association between macular degeneration and high blood pressure (*hypertension*) and elevated cholesterol levels.

Research has shown that people with controlled hypertension (below 160/95) are twice as likely to develop macular degeneration as people with healthy blood pressure. For people with uncontrolled hypertension (above 160/95), the risk is three times greater than for people with normal blood pressure. Hypertension has also been linked with an increased risk for wet macular degeneration and a more rapid progression of the disease.

Abnormal cholesterol levels may also be associated with an increased risk for macular degeneration. One study found that high cholesterol levels, coupled with high blood pressure, raised the risk for wet macular degeneration. At this time, it remains unclear exactly how cholesterol levels contribute to the disease.

Poor Nutrition

To understand why poor nutrition may increase the likelihood of getting macular degeneration, it is useful to know about *free radicals*. Free radicals are unstable, high-energy molecules in the body that can damage cells. Every second of every day, free radicals are being formed in the body as a result of digesting food and converting it to energy, of repairing injuries, and of thousands of other biochemical reactions. Full of energy, free radicals seek to react with other molecules in the body in order to release some of that energy. If they happen to meet up with a sensitive system within the body, such as our DNA (the genetic code that determines who we are), they can damage it.

Such damage contributes to many health disorders, including macular degeneration. Free radicals formed in the macula may damage sensitive tissues, tiny blood vessels, and other structures within the eye, increasing the likelihood that an individual will develop macular degeneration.

Antioxidants—disease-fighting substances found in fresh foods such as fruits and vegetables—are the body's natural defense system and help keep free radicals from damaging other molecules. Think of antioxidants as a giant wall stopping that snowball in its path. With a poor diet that is low in antioxidants, there is no wall, and the snowball continues to grow larger and race downhill faster.

Exposure to Sunlight

Long-term exposure to sunlight may be another risk factor for macular degeneration. Sunlight contains the colors of the rainbow—red, orange, yellow, green, blue, indigo, and violet. *Blue light*, which includes blue, indigo, and violet, contains the most energy. In animal studies, scientists have found that blue light damages retinal cells. This has led them to believe that blue light may be involved in the onset or worsening of macular degeneration. People who spend a lot of time outdoors are encouraged to use protective eyewear to reduce exposure to harmful light and also to check their vision regularly for signs of macular degeneration.

Existing Macular Degeneration

It may seem obvious, but having macular degeneration is considered a risk factor for the disease. If you have the dry or wet form of the disease in one eye, that increases the likelihood of getting it in the other eye. For example, if you have wet macular degeneration in one eye, you have a 20 to 30 percent chance of developing the wet form in the other eye within three to five years.

Similarly, having dry macular degeneration means you have a greater chance of developing advanced dry macular degeneration. And having advanced dry macular degeneration raises the risk of developing the wet form of the condition.

Does Cataract Surgery Cause Macular Degeneration?

A *cataract* is a clouding of the lens of the eye that develops slowly and can be treated with surgery. For years, people have been asking if having cataracts or undergoing cataract surgery leads to macular degeneration. The answer is likely no. Because cataracts, like macular degeneration, tend to occur with advancing age, it is not uncommon for elderly people to have both of these conditions. Recent research, however, suggests that these two eye diseases usually develop independently of each other.

In the 1970s and 1980s, it was thought that cataract surgery may result in the acceleration of macular degeneration. Since that time, several advances in cataract surgery have occurred. For example, the *intraocular lenses* used today have ultraviolet (UV) light filters that help protect the macula. In addition, cataract surgery is now less invasive, takes less time, and results in less inflammation. For these reasons, it is unlikely that modern cataract surgery plays a major role in the development or progression of macular degeneration. However, for people with wet macular degeneration and visually significant cataracts, it is recommended that the macular degeneration be stabilized with treatment before cataract surgery is performed.

In Summary

- Macular degeneration is most common in people over age fifty, and age is the greatest risk factor for the disease.
- Macular degeneration affects central vision, which is required for activities such as reading and driving.
- There are two basic types of macular degeneration: dry macular degeneration and wet macular degeneration.
- Dry macular degeneration typically progresses slowly and may not produce noticeable symptoms.
- Wet macular degeneration can progress rapidly and may result in significant visual impairment.

- Having macular degeneration in one eye increases the likelihood of developing it in the other eye.
- Having cataract surgery is unlikely to increase the risk for macular degeneration.

Gaining an understanding of macular degeneration can play an important role in preventing the disease from progressing and, thus, in preserving eyesight.

2 Symptoms and Signs of Macular Degeneration

A number of symptoms and signs are associated with macular degeneration, but many people ignore them or mistake them for symptoms and signs of other eye conditions. In these cases, people often wait too long before seeking treatment for this vision-threatening condition. This is unfortunate, because with early treatment, there is a greater chance of slowing the progression of the disease, preserving good vision, or even improving vision. Being aware of the symptoms and signs of macular degeneration and seeking treatment *immediately* if you notice any changes in your vision are critical for preserving your eyesight.

Early Symptoms of Dry Macular Degeneration

In the earliest stages of dry macular degeneration, you may have no symptoms. When symptoms do develop, they may include:

- blurred vision
- decreased central vision
- small blank spots in or near the central field of vision
- mild, chronic distortion of central vision

Early Symptoms of Macular Degeneration

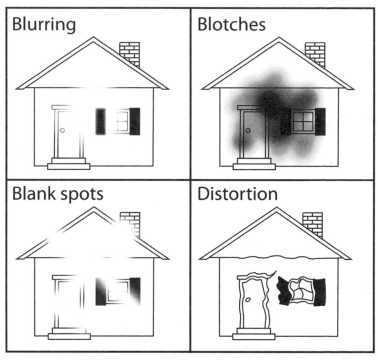

These illustrations represent the types of early symptoms that are common with macular degeneration: blurring, blotches, blank spots, and distortion.

Although you may not be aware that your vision is changing, you may notice that:

- you require brighter lighting to read
- you require brighter lighting to perform your daily activities
- objects do not seem as bright or as colorful as they used to

With dry macular degeneration, changes usually affect the central field of vision and not the peripheral vision. Many individuals mistakenly assume that these symptoms signal nothing more than a need for a new prescription for their eyeglasses. Others write them off as signs of cataracts (clouding of the lens of the eye).

Progression of Dry Macular Degeneration

Symptoms of dry macular degeneration typically progress slowly over a period of months or years. Blurring may become more pronounced, reading or other close work may become more difficult, distance vision may worsen, and areas in the central field of vision may blur or darken completely. In some cases, as dry macular degeneration progresses, patients begin to experience mild, chronic distortion. If the distortion worsens rapidly, this is usually a sign that dry macular degeneration has developed into wet macular degeneration.

Early Symptoms of Wet Macular Degeneration

In the early stages of wet macular degeneration, when abnormal blood vessels begin to grow, you may not experience any symptoms initially. When symptoms do surface, they may include:

- distortion or "waviness" of straight lines in the central field of vision
- blurred vision
- blank spots
- blotches
- smudging
- objects appearing less bright or less colorful

The most common early sign of wet macular degeneration is distortion in the central field of vision. When looking at objects that have straight lines— such as the edges of a door, the edges of miniblinds on a window, or the sides of a television set—the lines appear wavy or crooked.

In the early stages, any blurring, blank spots, blotches, or smudges affect only central vision—not peripheral vision. These warning signs may be most noticeable when looking at someone's face, watching a television show, or reading a book. You may find that you have to move your head to the side or tilt it up or down to see clearly.

Progression of Wet Macular Degeneration

Although the symptoms of wet macular degeneration may be subtle at first, they usually progress rapidly and become more pronounced over a period of days or weeks, or sometimes months. Straight lines become more distorted or wavy. Blurring intensifies. Blank spots, blotches, and smudges become larger or more pronounced. Objects may appear to have lost most or all of their brightness or color.

In cases in which severe macular degeneration has reduced the vision in both eyes, patients may experience visual hallucinations, or "phantom" images. As mentioned earlier, this condition is known as Charles Bonnet syndrome. These phantom images can be very clear in detail and may take the shape of patterns, lines, buildings, landscapes, animals, faces, and more. How does this happen? Basically, it is the mind trying to interpret what the eyes are seeing, by filling in any visual blank spots with images stored in the memory. Phantom images may be fleeting or may last for hours; they may be in vivid color or in stark black-and-white. These images can be quite alarming, especially when they first begin to occur. Turning lights on or off, closing your eyes, or moving your eyes from side to side may make any bothersome images disappear.

Self-Testing

Several simple do-it-yourself tests can help detect symptoms of macular degeneration. Performing these self-tests on a regular basis can alert you to changes in your vision that may be signs of early macular degeneration or indications that the disease is progressing. In addition to being easy to use, these self-testing methods are free and readily available.

Amsler Grid

One of the best ways to test your vision for signs of macular degeneration is by using the *Amsler grid*. Basically, the Amsler grid looks like a sheet of graph paper with a dark dot in the center. To use it, simply hold the grid in one hand about fourteen inches from your eyes. Close one eye, cover it with the palm of your other hand, and then focus on the dot in the center with your open eye. (If you normally wear glasses for reading, be sure to wear them when you test your eyes with the Amsler grid.) As you stare at the central dot, notice if any of the lines on the grid appear distorted or wavy, or if any of the lines or squares seem to blur, fade, or disappear. Put the grid

Amsler Grid

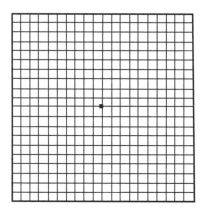

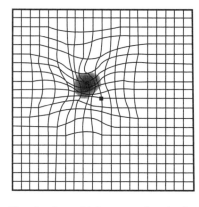

The Amsler grid is a test for checking yourself for symptoms of macular degeneration. The top grid represents normal vision. The bottom grid represents distortion of central vision, which is an early symptom of macular degeneration.

down, uncover your eye, and focus on something other than the grid for a few seconds. Then test your other eye in the same way.

If you are diagnosed with macular degeneration, it is recommended that you test your eyes with the Amsler grid on a daily basis. The Amsler grid provides a good baseline to help you detect changes in your vision. If you do notice any changes, inform your eye care professional immediately.

It is a good idea to mark any areas of concern on your Amsler grid. Simply mark any spots that appear different, and write down what the problem is, such as distortion, wavy lines, blurring, blank spots, blotches, or smudges. Keeping a record of current areas of distortion, blurring, or blank spots in this manner can be helpful in tracking progression of the disease. If the areas change in any way, such as becoming larger or more pronounced, bring it to the attention of your eye care specialist. Similarly, take note if any areas of concern appear to move to a different portion of the grid. Remember to take your Amsler grid with you to your eye appointment. To download a copy of the grid from the Internet, visit www.amd.org or www.macula.org. You will also find the grid in the appendix of this book.

Outdoor Self-Tests

Almost any time you are outside, you have an opportunity to test your vision for early signs of macular degeneration. Simply look out into the distance, and focus on an object with straight lines, such as a building, telephone pole, or street sign. Close one eye, cover it with the palm of your hand, and then check for any signs of distortion, wavy lines, blurring, or blank spots with your open eye.

Indoor Self-Tests

You can also test your eyes in the setting of your home. Windowpanes, miniblinds, and the edges of doors make ideal test subjects because they have straight lines. As with the other self-tests, test one eye at a time by closing and covering the other eye and taking note of any distortion, waviness, blurring, or blank spots.

Reading offers another excellent way to test your vision. In fact, you can test your vision with this book right now. Simply focus on the center of the page, and testing one eye at a time, check for any blurring, blank spots, smudges, or lines of print that look wavy. Look at the edge of the page, and take note of any distortion or wavy lines. Report any problems to your eye care professional immediately.

Importance of Early Detection

It is common for macular degeneration patients to report having "good days" and "bad days" with their vision. On good days, their vision seems more normal. On bad days, their symptoms appear to worsen. The changes in vision may be due to lighting conditions, overall health changes, or changes in the amount of leakage under the retina.

The problem with having good days and bad days is that it often makes people who have not yet been diagnosed with the disease delay seeking treatment. When bad days occur, they may consider calling an eye care specialist for an appointment. But then, when they have a good day, they may write off that bad day as a temporary problem that simply went away on its own. If you are experiencing good days and bad days with your vision, do not hesitate to schedule an appointment with your eye care specialist.

It cannot be stressed enough how critical it is to detect wet macular degeneration early and before much damage has occurred. With treatment at the earliest stages, the chances are much better that severe vision loss can be prevented. In some cases, early detection and treatment may even improve vision. That is why it is so important to know the symptoms and signs of macular degeneration, to test your vision regularly, and to seek specialized care immediately if you notice any changes in your vision.

In Summary

- Symptoms of macular degeneration include blurred vision and blank spots.
- Distortion is one of the most common symptoms of wet macular degeneration.
- Checking your eyes with simple self-tests on a regular basis can help you detect symptoms of macular degeneration.
- People often wait too long before seeing an eye doctor for macular degeneration.
- Delaying treatment may result in vision loss.
- Early detection is key. Seek treatment immediately if you notice any changes in your vision.

Being aware of the symptoms and signs of macular degeneration and seeking treatment immediately for them may help prevent vision loss due to this disease.

3 Getting a Diagnosis

To accurately diagnose macular degeneration, an eye care specialist will take many factors into consideration and may perform a variety of diagnostic tests. It is a good idea to become familiar with the various types of tests used to diagnose macular degeneration. Knowing what to expect from your consultation will help you be prepared so that you can make the most of your time with your eye care specialist.

Choosing an Eye Care Specialist

When choosing an eye care specialist for your eye examination, it is helpful to understand the types of eye care providers. These include *optometrists, general ophthalmologists,* and *retinal specialists.* Optometrists and general ophthalmologists specialize in general eye care, while retinal specialists are experts in diagnosing and treating macular degeneration and other problems related to the retina.

Optometrists

An optometrist, also called an optometric doctor (O.D.), specializes in general eye care. To become an optometrist, a person must first earn a college degree and then successfully complete four years of training at a special school for optometry. After obtaining a license to practice, an optometrist typically performs routine eye exams, prescribes eyeglasses and contact lenses for vision correction, and in some instances, prescribes medication for certain medical conditions of the eye. In most states, optometrists are not licensed to perform major treatments or surgery. If you visit an optometrist for an eye exam, and macular degeneration is suspected, you may be advised to make an appointment with a general ophthalmologist or a retinal specialist for further evaluation.

General Ophthalmologists

A general ophthalmologist is a licensed medical doctor who has earned a bachelor's degree, completed medical school, and earned a doctor of medicine degree (M.D.). An ophthalmologist must then complete at least four years of additional training in ophthalmology. After obtaining a medical license, an ophthalmologist is able to perform eye surgery as well as provide general eye care. These eye care physicians typically specialize in certain types of eye surgery, such as cataract surgery, corneal surgery (such as laser refractive surgery, or LASIK), or retinal surgery. If a general ophthalmologist sees signs of macular degeneration during your eye exam, you may be referred to a retinal specialist for further testing and treatment.

Retinal Specialists

Retinal specialists are ophthalmologists who typically undergo two additional years of extensive training after obtaining their ophthalmology certificate. They are highly trained in the diagnosis and treatment of retinal problems, including macular degeneration and diabetic retinopathy. (*Retinopathy* is the term used to describe a "diseased" retina.) A retinal specialist uses advanced examination and imaging tools to evaluate the health of the macula and the retina in great detail. This helps with establishing the diagnosis and determining treatment options for macular degeneration.

Preparing for Your Eye Examination

To get the most out of your consultation, be prepared. Your eye care professional will want to know about your medical and vision history, so gather your medical records and take them with you to your appointment. Specifically, your eye doctor will want to know about:

- any past or present health conditions
- any surgical procedures
- any past or present eye disorders, injuries, or operations
- all medications you are currently taking, including prescription medications, over-the-counter remedies, vitamins, supplements, herbs, and homeopathic products (which is important because some drugs can affect vision)
- past or present smoking

- past or present alcohol consumption
- any family history of medical problems or eye conditions
- your primary care doctor's name and contact information

Your eye care specialist will also want to know about the history of your current symptoms, so take a little time prior to your appointment to jot down:

- any symptoms or changes in your vision that you are currently experiencing
- the approximate date when you first noticed these symptoms or changes in your vision
- whether the symptoms occur intermittently, occur only in certain environments (such as when lights are dim), or are present all the time
- whether the symptoms have remained steady or appear to be worsening

Be sure to take your eyeglasses—distance and reading glasses if you use both—or contact lenses to your consultation. Take your sunglasses, too, because your doctor will probably use eyedrops to dilate your pupils, which can make your eyes sensitive to bright light. It is prudent to arrange for someone to drive you home.

Your Eye Examination

A routine eye examination may be as brief as half an hour, but a comprehensive exam for the diagnosis of macular degeneration may take two hours or longer. The length of your exam will depend on

Snellen Eye Chart

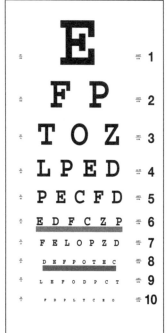

Eye care professionals use the Snellen eye chart to test visual acuity. It is usually read from a distance of 20 feet.

several factors, including which diagnostic tests are performed.

Visual Acuity Testing

Visual acuity refers to the clarity of your central vision, or simply put, how well you see. Visual acuity testing measures central vision, which is commonly affected by macular degeneration. With all of the high-tech diagnostic tools available to eye doctors today, the tool most commonly used to test visual acuity is decidedly low-tech—it's the Snellen visual acuity chart, the basic eye chart developed in the nineteenth century.

Visual acuity is expressed by phrases such as "20/20" and "20/40." Most people have heard these phrases but may not understand what they mean. In the United States, the first "20" stands for 20 feet, which is the distance you are from the eye chart while being tested. Since most examination rooms are not 20 feet long, a mirror is used to achieve the optical distance of 20 feet. The second number in the phrase indicates how much your visual acuity differs from the norm. For example, if you have 20/20 vision—which is considered ideal for a healthy person—you are able to identify objects or letters that a person with normal eyesight can identify from 20 feet away. If your vision is 20/40, this indicates that what people with good vision can identify from 40 feet away must be brought to 20 feet in front of you in order for you to be able to identify it. The higher the second number, the worse your visual acuity.

When checking your visual acuity, your eye care specialist will test each eye separately. It is common for one eye to have better visual acuity than the other. As your eye care specialist tests your visual acuity, be sure to indicate if you are seeing any wavy lines, blurring, or blank spots, which may be signs of macular degeneration.

Eye Pressure Testing

Testing the pressure inside the eyes is commonly performed to screen for *glaucoma*, a condition that causes damage to the optic nerve (the nerve of the eye). Your eye care professional may use one of a number of methods to test *eye pressure.*

In one commonly used method called Goldman tonometry, a drop of yellow *fluorescein* dye and topical anesthetic is put in your eye, and you are then asked to place your chin on the chin rest of a device called a *slit lamp.* A slit lamp is a modified microscope, with a bright light, that allows an eye care specialist to view the eye under high magnification. The prism head of a small, spring-loaded pressure sensor is gently placed against the *tear film* on the surface of your eyeball, and the pressure reading is done under blue light, which illuminates the dye.

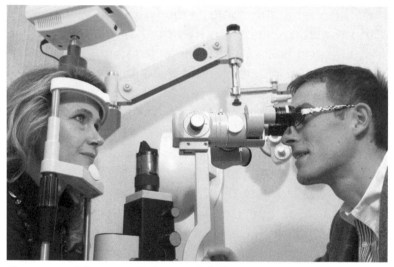

Eye care specialists use a slit lamp, with high-intensity light, to examine the inner structures of the eye.

Nowadays, many doctors use a newer device called a *Tono-Pen,* which looks like a pen, to measure eye pressure. With this method, an anesthetic eyedrop is used to numb the surface of your eye. The tip of the Tono-Pen is then gently placed against the eye's tear film, and a digital readout displays the eye pressure measurement.

With both of these methods, the eyes are tested individually. If eye pressure is high, you may be at risk for glaucoma in the affected eye(s). High eye pressure is not considered a sign of macular degeneration.

Visual Field Testing

Visual field refers to peripheral vision. As mentioned previously, peripheral vision is your "side vision," or your ability to see objects that are not in your direct line of vision. A visual field test is performed as you look at a small, central point while lights of various sizes are projected at various locations away from that central point. You are asked to indicate each time you see the light. In general, peripheral vision is not affected by macular degeneration. Therefore, a visual field test is not a routine test for macular degeneration.

Test for Range of Eye Movement

The *range of eye movement* is not used specifically to diagnose macular degeneration, but it is generally part of a comprehensive eye exam. Although the test for range of eye movement does not involve any high-tech equipment, it does give your eye care professional valuable information about the condition of your eye muscles. Testing one eye first, then the other, and then the two eyes together, your eye doctor will have you look upward, downward, and from side to side while he or she shines a light or holds an object in front of you and asks you to "follow" it.

Amsler Grid Test

When checking for macular degeneration, your eye care specialist will test your eyes using the Amsler grid. As noted in the previous chapter, the Amsler grid looks like a sheet of graph paper with a dark dot in the center. You will be asked to cover one eye and focus the open eye on the dot in the center of the grid. If any of the lines on the grid appear distorted, wavy, blurry, or blank, it may be an indication of macular degeneration.

Dilation of the Pupils

As part of a comprehensive eye examination, your eye care specialist may *dilate*, or widen, your pupils using eyedrops. Dilating the pupils provides the doctor with a better view of the internal structures of the eye—particularly, the macula and the peripheral retina. It usually takes thirty minutes or more for the eyedrops to take full effect. After the pupils are fully dilated, the doctor may use a variety of sophisticated tools to examine the eye.

Dilation of the pupils often makes your vision blurred and your eyes sensitive to bright light. The effects of dilating eyedrops take about three to four hours to wear off.

Examination of the Front of the Eye

To examine the structures of the front of the eye, your eye care specialist will use a slit lamp. For this test, you will be seated comfortably at the slit lamp and asked to rest your chin and forehead on supports. Using the slit lamp, the doctor can examine the following parts of the front of the eye:

- *Eyelids:* The eyelids will be examined for any signs of infection or malfunction.
- *Conjunctiva:* This is the thin, transparent membrane that covers the white part of the eye as well as the inner surface of the eyelid. The doctor will check this area for evidence of inflammation, which can cause the white part of the eye to appear red and irritated. When inflammation is present, it is often a sign of allergy or infection.

- *Cornea:* The cornea is the clear, dome-shaped front surface of the eye. It does most of the focusing work for the eye. When examining the cornea, the doctor will look for signs of inflammation, irritation, or infection.
- *Tear film:* The tear film is a protective liquid layer lubricating the conjunctiva and the cornea. It creates a smooth surface for light to pass through. With age, the tear film loses its ability to adequately lubricate the eye. This condition is called *dry eye*, but it has no relationship to dry macular degeneration.
- *Iris:* The iris is the part of the eye that appears to have color. The iris controls the size of the pupil—reducing it in bright light and enlarging it in low light—to regulate the amount of light coming into the eye. Your eye care specialist will check the appearance of the iris and test it to see if it responds correctly to light.
- *Anterior chamber:* Separating the cornea and the iris is a clear, fluid-filled space called the anterior chamber. The doctor will check this area for signs of infection, inflammation, or hemorrhage.
- *Lens:* The eye's lens works with the cornea to focus images. The doctor will check the lens for signs of clouding, which indicates the presence of a cataract. Because cataracts can significantly impair vision, it is important to check for this condition when you are experiencing vision problems. Be aware that it is possible to have cataracts *and* macular degeneration at the same time.

Examination of the Back of the Eye

Viewing the back of the eye is a critical part of your examination because the structures damaged by macular degeneration are located in this area. *Ophthalmoscopy* is a test that allows your eye care specialist to view the structures at the back of the eye—including the retina, choroid, blood vessels, and *optic disk*—under magnification. The optic disk, located a the back of the retina, is also called the "blind spot" because there are no photoreceptors in this area. This test is usually performed while your pupils are dilated.

There are two commonly used techniques for ophthalmoscopy. The first technique involves the combined use of a slit lamp and a viewing lens for a detailed, high-magnification examination of the macula and the optic nerve. The second technique utilizes a special headset light and a handheld magnifier that allows your doctor to see the peripheral retina and an overview of the macula and optic nerve. Your doctor may use one or both of these techniques, depending on the circumstances. Usually, ophthalmoscopy allows the doctor to examine the following:

- *Vitreous gel:* This clear, jellylike substance occupying the area between the lens and the retina is checked for signs of hemorrhage, inflammation, and liquefaction. Vitreous hemorrhage is an uncommon complication of macular degeneration.
- *Peripheral retina:* Although the peripheral, or outer, portion of the retina is usually not affected by macular degeneration, your eye

care specialist will check it because it can be involved in a number of other eye disorders that may affect vision, such as retinal tear or detachment.

- *Optic nerve:* The optic nerve is like a cable that connects the eye to the brain. Macular degeneration typically does not affect the optic nerve, but your doctor will examine this area because damage to it can be a cause of vision problems.
- *Macula:* The macula is the center part of the retina and is critical for central vision. Because the macula is the principal part of the eye affected by macular degeneration, your doctor will pay special attention to this area during an exam. Specifically, the doctor will be looking for signs of dry or wet macular degeneration.

Signs of Dry Macular Degeneration Include:

- drusen, which appear as yellow deposits
- changes in pigmentation of the macula, including a mottled or uneven appearance
- atrophy, or thinning, of the macula

Signs of Wet Macular Degeneration Include:

- subretinal blood, which is blood that has accumulated under the retina
- other subretinal fluids, which are fluids other than blood that have accumulated under the retina
- lipid deposits, which are fatty deposits within or under the retina

- retinal thickening, which may be due to the accumulation of blood and/or other fluids within the retinal tissue
- disciform scarring, also called *fibrosis*, under the retina, which indicates irreversible damage

Fundus Fluorescein Angiography

To make an accurate diagnosis of macular degeneration, your eye care specialist may recommend a test called *fundus fluorescein angiography*. The fundus of the eye is the interior surface of the eye, opposite the lens.

In this procedure, which is usually performed with the pupils dilated, fluorescein dye is injected into a vein in your arm. The dye travels through the bloodstream, and when it reaches the retina, a special high-speed camera takes a series of photographs of the retina. The images produced in this test can help your retinal specialist identify changes in pigmentation, abnormal blood vessels, and any leakage in the retina.

Fundus fluorescein angiography can be especially important in getting an accurate diagnosis of macular degeneration because it can rule out many other conditions that affect the retina, the macula, and your vision and that mimic macular degeneration. These other conditions have different characteristics when viewed with fluorescein angiography. With this test, your doctor can accurately determine whether or not you have macular degeneration.

Optical Coherence Tomography

Optical coherence tomography (*OCT*) is a non invasive test that is commonly performed when macular degeneration is suspected. OCT uses light technology to produce a scan of the macula. The scan shows a cross-sectional image of the retina that allows the doctor to judge the thickness of the retina, to see if the shape of the macula is normal or abnormal, to identify the presence of fluid, and to determine if leakage has resulted in the buildup of fluid under the macula or within the retina. OCT is an excellent tool for diagnosing and monitoring macular degeneration.

An OCT machine is similar to a slit lamp. The OCT technician will ask you to place your chin in a chin rest and look straight into the machine as it takes the scan. An OCT evaluation takes about 15 minutes.

Stages of Macular Degeneration

When making a diagnosis of macular degeneration, your eye care specialist will inform you about the type and possible stage of the disease. Dry macular degeneration has three stages—early, intermediate, and advanced—based on the extent of degenerative changes in one or both of your eyes. Note that if you are diagnosed with macular degeneration in both eyes, it is possible that each eye will be at a different stage.

Early Stage

In the early stage of the disease, the most common finding is the presence of drusen (mounds of waste products, or debris) on the macula. Typically, at this stage, the drusen are small. In the earliest stage, there is usually no noticeable impairment of vision.

Intermediate Stage

By the time the disease reaches the intermediate stage, the drusen have usually increased to medium size. At this stage, you may start to notice changes in your vision, such as blurring, needing more light for reading or doing detail work, blank spots, or mild distortion.

Advanced Stage

Evidence that may indicate dry macular degeneration has progressed to the advanced stage includes:

- large drusen
- pigment changes in the retina
- geographic atrophy, which includes a break-down in the light-sensitive cells, retinal pigment epithelium (RPE) cells, and choroidal capillaries of the macula

In this stage, problems with central vision are more pronounced. The development of abnormal blood vessels under the retina indicates the onset of wet macular degeneration, which is considered an advanced stage of dry macular degeneration.

Fundus Fluorescein Angiography

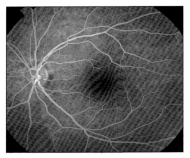 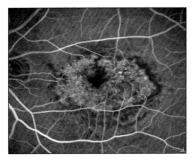

A normal eye after a fluorescein angiography. The test uses a special dye and camera to examine the blood flow to the retina and the blood vessels under it.

The fluorescein angiography above shows an eye of a patient with wet macular degeneration. Tiny blood vessels are leaking under the macula.

Optical Coherence Tomography (OCT)

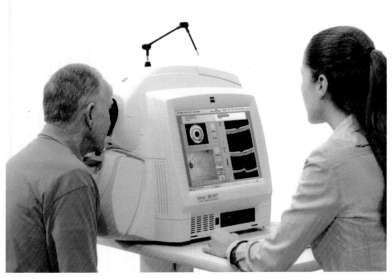

Optical coherence tomography (OCT) is like a CT scan of the macula. The scan uses light technology to map changes in the macula. *Photo courtesy of Carl Zeiss Meditec, Inc.*

Optical Coherence Tomography
Normal Macula

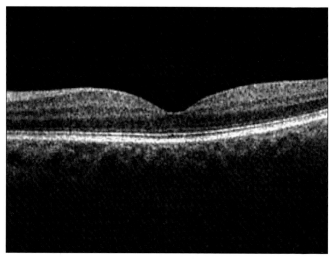

This OCT scan shows a smooth, normal macula. The macula is located in the central part of the retina.

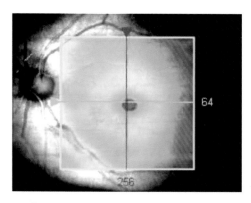

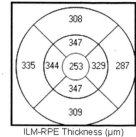

ILM-RPE Thickness (µm)

In this OCT scan the normal macula is shown by the smooth green and yellow colors. The numerical map on the right tells the ophthalmologist the thickness of the macula in micrometers.

Optical Coherence Tomography
Dry Macular Degeneration

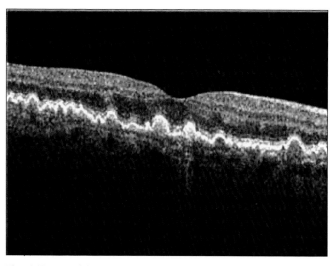

This OCT scan of dry macular degeneration shows multiple deposits (drusen) under the macula. There are no fluid cavities.

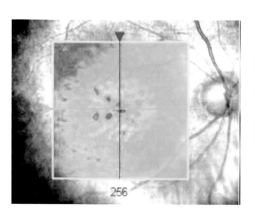

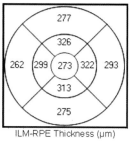

ILM-RPE Thickness (μm)

In this image from the same OCT scan, the green shows a normal thickness of the macula; the yellow shows a slight thickening of the macula. The numerical map to the right represents the thickness of the macula.

Optical Coherence Tomography
Wet Macular Degeneration

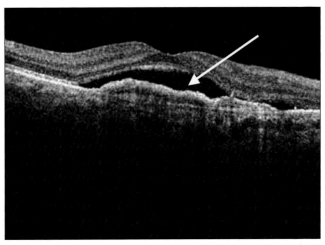

In the OCT scan above, the arrow shows a build-up of fluid under the macula.

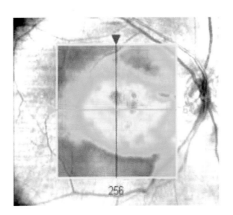

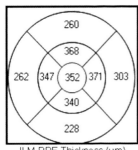

ILM-RPE Thickness (µm)

In this map of wet macular degeneration, the yellow and red areas show thickening and elevation of the macula. The numerical map to the right shows the thickness of the macula.

Questions to Ask Your Eye Care Specialist

When you are given a diagnosis of macular degeneration, it is normal to have questions. Here are some questions you may want to ask your eye care specialist:

- Do I have macular degeneration in one or both eyes?
- What type and stage of macular degeneration do I have?
- How will I know if the disease is progressing?
- Are there any symptoms or signs I should be aware of that would require immediate treatment?
- What treatment do you recommend?
- Are there any lifestyle changes you would suggest?
- Are there any support groups you would recommend?
- Are there any tools or products that might be helpful for me?
- Are there things I can do to help with the treatment/management of my macular degeneration?

Coping Emotionally

When you or a loved one is diagnosed with macular degeneration, it can stir up a lot of emotions. This is completely understandable. When you consider how much we rely on our vision in our everyday lives, it's easy to see how a diagnosis of this vision-threatening disease can be devastating. The possibility of a loss of independence can be particularly disturbing.

When faced with a diagnosis of macular degeneration, some people adjust to their new way of life with relative ease, others experience a temporary sense of sadness, and still others develop full-blown depression. The way you react to the news depends on many factors, including the degree of your vision loss, your age at diagnosis, your lifestyle at diagnosis, and even your general personality and the level of support you have from family and friends. If you find that you are having trouble adjusting or that feelings of sadness persist, talk to your eye care specialist about your feelings. Your doctor can refer you to a professional who can help.

In Summary

- Make an appointment with an eye care specialist if you are experiencing any symptoms of macular degeneration.
- If macular degeneration is suspected by your optometrist or ophthalmologist, you may be referred to a retinal specialist.
- A comprehensive eye exam will include a variety of diagnostic tests to examine the front and back portions of the eye.
- When macular degeneration is suspected, a noninvasive test called optical coherence tomography is commonly performed. This is a high-resolution scan of your macula.
- In some cases, a diagnostic test called fundus fluorescein angiography may be recommended in order to diagnose wet macular degeneration.

- If you are diagnosed with macular degeneration, ask what type of the disease you have: wet or dry. If you are diagnosed with dry macular degeneration, ask what stage: early, intermediate, or advanced.
- Understand that being diagnosed with macular degeneration may have an emotional impact on you.

Knowing what to expect from the eye examination process can help you feel more comfortable when seeking a diagnosis for symptoms associated with macular degeneration.

4 Treatments for Macular Degeneration

With macular degeneration, the goal of treatment has traditionally been to manage the disease by slowing its progress. In years past, doctors could only hope to delay vision loss—there was no prospect of halting or reversing it. In recent years, however, treating macular degeneration has been an area of intense research by doctors and scientists. As a result, the scientific community has made major advances in the development of treatment options for wet macular degeneration, which progresses rapidly and may cause significant vision loss. Although there is still no cure for the disease, the possibility of stabilizing or even restoring vision now exists.

Work is also ongoing to develop treatments for dry macular degeneration, which progresses gradually and does not usually cause severe vision loss. Currently, the treatment of dry macular degeneration focuses on reducing the risk for progression to more advanced stages, including conversion to the wet form of the disease.

Managing Dry Macular Degeneration

Current management of dry macular degeneration focuses on detecting the disease early and preventing its progression. Many people who are diagnosed with the disease have few or no symptoms. Although serious vision loss may occur with dry macular degeneration, it typically takes many years to do so. Severe vision loss can occur when dry macular degeneration turns into wet macular degeneration. However, dry macular degeneration does not always turn into the wet form of the disease.

Many people with this disease are frustrated by the lack of a cure. Some people worry that their condition will worsen, and they feel as if there is nothing they can do to stop it. However, although there are no specific treatments for dry macular degeneration, there are things you can do to manage it and reduce the rate of progression.

As with many other medical conditions, paying attention to diet and other lifestyle issues can allow you to take an active role in disease prevention and progression. For example, studies funded by the U.S. National Institutes of Health (NIH) have found that consuming certain antioxidants can decrease the risk of developing advanced macular degeneration. Monitoring your own eye health is another useful measure.

Vitamins and Nutritional Supplements

To decrease the chance of your dry macular degeneration worsening, your eye care professional may recommend that you take specific doses of certain vitamins and nutritional supplements. Funded by the

NIH, the *Age-Related Eye Disease Study* (*AREDS*), which followed 3,600 individuals with different stages of macular degeneration, found that taking high levels of antioxidants, zinc, and copper reduced the risk of developing advanced macular degeneration by about 25 percent in patients with moderate dry macular degeneration. The specific daily doses used for this study were:

- vitamin C—500 milligrams
- vitamin E—400 International Units
- beta-carotene—15 milligrams (equivalent to 25,000 International Units of vitamin A)
- zinc—80 milligrams
- copper—2 milligrams

Your doctor can tell you if these vitamins and supplements are right for you. If the AREDS formulation is recommended for you, be sure to review all vitamins and nutritional supplements you are currently taking with your doctor first. Note that if you are a smoker, you should not take the AREDS formulation, since beta-carotene in the form of vitamin A has been found to increase the risk of lung cancer in smokers. If you are a smoker and have dry macular degeneration, talk to your doctor about other options.

Scientists are continuing to investigate whether other vitamins and supplements may be effective in the management, or possibly even the prevention, of dry macular degeneration. Two of the supplements being studied are the antioxidant *lutein* (found in certain fruits and vegetables) and omega-3 fatty acids (commonly available in the form of fish oil). Talk to your eye care professional before taking these supplements.

Monitoring at Home

Your doctor may also give you a small Amsler grid to take home with you. This simple device allows you to check for changes in your condition at home. It consists of straight lines in a grid pattern, with a small, dark dot in the center. Because macular degeneration distorts the retina, changes can manifest themselves as distortion or bending of the grid lines.

As noted previously, when using the grid, be sure to wear your reading glasses and have good lighting. Hold the grid in one hand at a comfortable reading distance, about fourteen inches away. Close one eye and cover it with your other hand; then look at the central dot and check that all the lines are straight and all the squares are of the same size. Then check your other eye.

Your doctor will recommend that you use the grid on a daily basis. If the lines become more distorted, blurred, or discolored, consult your doctor immediately.

Managing Wet Macular Degeneration

Although there is still no cure for wet macular degeneration, great strides have been made in the management of the disease. Vision loss in wet macular degeneration is associated with abnormal blood vessels that grow under the retina and can cause swelling or bleeding. Modern treatments use drugs that target these blood vessels. The use of these drugs has made treatment for wet macular degeneration less invasive and introduced the possibility of preventing further vision loss in a majority of patients and improving vision in some.

Techniques used to treat wet macular degeneration are aimed at stopping or slowing the growth of the abnormal blood vessels under the retina. They are also designed to halt or reduce the leakage of blood or other fluids associated with these abnormal blood vessels. Although these treatments can be effective, they do not provide permanent relief from wet macular degeneration and typically require ongoing management.

Drug Injections

The most common and effective treatment for wet macular degeneration today involves an injection of medication into the affected eye. As noted above, wet macular degeneration occurs when abnormal blood vessels grow under the retina. These blood vessels require a substance called vascular endothelial growth factor (VEGF) to survive. Drugs known as anti-VEGF agents target this substance and cause the abnormal blood vessels to shrink.

As a matter of historical perspective, the first anti-VEGF drugs developed were initially used to fight cancer. Cancer cells also require abnormal blood vessels in order to grow and reproduce. Anti-VEGF drugs can help fight cancer by shrinking these blood vessels and depriving the cancer of its blood supply. However, these drugs are not considered chemotherapy drugs.

Fortunately, scientists realized that tiny doses of anti-VEGF drugs were safe and effective in fighting wet macular degeneration, as well. Initial studies published in 2005 confirmed that injecting these drugs into the eyeball was highly effective in reducing the leakage associated with wet macular degeneration. Since then, this treatment method has become increasingly common.

If your retinal specialist recommends this type of treatment, one of the following anti-VEGF drugs may be injected into your eyeball. These drugs work in a similar manner to shrink abnormal blood vessels.

- *Lucentis (ranibizumab):* Lucentis is FDA-approved for the treatment of wet macular degeneration. Initial clinical trials for Lucentis showed that it slowed leakage and stabilized vision in about 90 percent of people. What is even more encouraging is that vision improved for about one-third of the people in the original studies.

- *Avastin (bevacizumab):* Avastin is widely used for the treatment of wet macular degeneration. Avastin was originally FDA-approved for colon cancer therapy. (When doctors use a drug to treat a disease that it was not initially designed to treat, it is called "off-label" usage. This is a very common practice with drugs that have been shown to be an effective treatment for other diseases.)

    A study sponsored by the National Eye Institute (part of the NIH) found Lucentis and Avastin to be equally effective in treating wet macular degeneration. Called the *Comparison of Age-Related Macular Degeneration Treatment Trial* (*CATT*), this study also found no major differences between the two drugs in terms of side effects. Serious, systemic side effects are very rare with either Lucentis or Avastin.

- *Eylea* (*aflibercept*): a newer drug, was approved by the FDA for treating wet macular degeneration in 2011. This drug belongs to a group of drugs called VEGF-Trap that work by blocking the substances that stimulate abnormal blood vessel growth. The FDA recommends monthly injections for the first three months and then monthly injections thereafter.

- *Macugen* (*pegaptanib sodium*): Macugen is FDA-approved for the treatment of wet macular degeneration. Studies show that it can significantly reduce the risk of vision loss in people with wet macular degeneration. However, in comparison to other anti-VEGF drugs, it is less likely to result in significant vision improvement. Because of this, Macugen is not used as commonly as often as other drugs.

Your retina specialist will discuss with you which drug is appropriate for you. He or she will also discuss how many injections you will need and how often they will be given. The frequency of your injections may be adjusted over time. For example, when Lucentis was first introduced, injections were given on a monthly basis for up to two years and then continued if the macular degeneration was still active. More-recent, large-scale clinical studies have shown that injections given on an "as-needed" basis are also effective. That is why most retinal specialists now tailor the number of injections and the interval between injections to a person's individual needs.

A commonly recommended course of initial treatment is approximately three injections given four to six weeks apart. After that, an eye examination is performed to evaluate whether or not macular degeneration is continuing to cause leakage of blood or other fluids in the retina. If this sign of active disease is noted, additional injections are given. If the leakage has stopped, the injections are halted until the leakage recurs. Most people need more than three injections to bring the leakage under control.

Once the leakage has stopped, regular eye exams (usually every one to three months) will be performed to detect any new or recurrent leakage. In most cases, leakage will eventually return, at which time injections will be resumed. In the early stages, if leakage recurs, you may not notice any symptoms. This is the reason for regular examinations. It is important to recognize any recurrence of leakage before too much damage occurs.

How Drug Injections Are Given

When treating wet macular degeneration with injectable drugs, your retinal specialist will inject the drug directly into the eyeball. Although this may seem frightening at first, rest assured that there is little or no discomfort; your eyeball is numbed before the injection, and the needles used are quite thin.

After your doctor has discussed the injection with you, he or she will begin to numb your eye. Anesthesia can be accomplished in a number of ways, including eyedrops, a numbing gel, or an injectable anesthetic given around the eye, very similar to what you might expect in a dentist's office. The numbing process takes about fifteen minutes.

After your eye is numb, your doctor will likely use a small instrument to hold your eyelids open so that you do not inadvertently blink during the injection. The surface of the eye is then disinfected with a few drops of antiseptic. It is normal to feel a mild burning sensation from the antiseptic. You may then be asked to look in a certain direction as your doctor administers the injection. The needle used is very small and is placed in a safe location in the white part of the eye. The actual injection will be completed in seconds, and your eye will then be rinsed.

Usually, there is no need for an eye patch following this treatment; in some cases, however, an eye patch may be used at the discretion of your doctor. You may also be prescribed antibiotic eyedrops to be used for a few days after the treatment. After this procedure, your eye may be irritated, sensitive to light, or teary, and you may experience temporary blurring of vision, so it is a good idea to have someone drive you home after the procedure.

Side Effects of Drug Injections

People most commonly experience mild irritation, such as a gritty or scratchy sensation, in the eye following an injection. Other common side effects include redness, blurred vision, and tearing. These side effects are usually mild and improve within a few days. Occasionally, people experience severe burning, but this typically resolves within a day. If severe burning or pain persists for more than one day, contact your retinal specialist immediately.

Hemorrhage on the white part of the eye (called the conjunctiva) may occur, but this typically goes away within two weeks and has no effect on vision. Occasionally, people have bloodstained tearing for a few days. Other side effects include floaters and increased eye pressure. Rare, but serious, side effects include retinal detachment, retinal tear, and infection.

You may have heard that anti-VEGF drugs, when given in high concentrations for the treatment of cancer, may be associated with an increased risk of high blood pressure, heart attack, or stroke. It is important to understand that when these drugs are used for cancer treatment, they are given intravenously in very high doses. In the treatment of wet macular degeneration, tiny doses of these drugs are used and are injected directly into the eyeball. These injections are typically not associated with side effects outside of the eye.

Photodynamic Therapy

Photodynamic therapy is another treatment that is sometimes used for wet macular degeneration. In the early 2000s, photodynamic therapy was the treatment of choice for wet macular degeneration. It was considered particularly useful for treating a subtype

Photodynamic Therapy

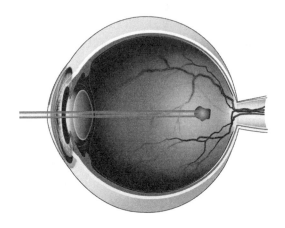

Photodynamic therapy involves the use of a drug called Visudyne, which is activated by a laser beam. The treatment destroys leaking blood vessels and helps reduce the risk of vision loss.

of wet macular degeneration—predominantly classic, in which the abnormal blood vessels rapidly leak blood or other fluids into the space under the retina.

Photodynamic therapy involves the use of a light-activated drug called Visudyne (verteporfin). Visudyne has a special affinity for the abnormal blood vessels that cause wet macular degeneration and concentrates in these blood vessels. A low-intensity, long-wavelength laser light is used to activate the drug, which then destroys the leaky blood vessels and inhibits the growth of new abnormal blood vessels. This laser light does not produce heat, which is why it is often referred to as a *cold laser*. Cold lasers are believed to target the abnormal blood vessels without affecting normal blood vessels or surrounding tissues the way high-intensity lasers do.

Clinical studies have shown that photodynamic therapy reduces the risk of vision loss by approximately 20 percent. It does not restore lost vision and usually does not improve vision. It is important to note that photodynamic therapy may cause minor damage to the retina.

Because anti-VEGF drugs have been shown to be more effective than photodynamic therapy, they have replaced photodynamic therapy as the treatment of choice for wet macular degeneration. However, in cases that are resistant to treatment with anti-VEGF drugs, a combination of anti-VEGF drug injections and photodynamic therapy may be used.

How Photodynamic Therapy Is Performed

For this treatment, you will first receive an infusion of Visudyne, which, as noted previously, activates in response to light of certain wavelengths. The infusion is administered into a vein in your arm over a period of ten to fifteen minutes. (Some patients may notice back pain during the infusion.) You will then be seated at a slit lamp, an instrument that allows the retinal specialist to see the retina and other structures of the back of the eye. You will be asked to rest your chin and forehead on supports.

A numbing eyedrop will be placed in your eye. Once the eye is numb, a special lens will be placed on the surface of the eye. This special lens allows the doctor to visualize the macula and also to target the area of interest for laser treatment. The cold laser light will then be focused on the macula and activated for eighty-one seconds.

The entire procedure takes about twenty minutes, and other than the minor discomfort of a needle stick in the arm, there is usually no pain associated with it.

Side Effects of Photodynamic Therapy

The vision in the treated eye may seem dark immediately following the treatment. This occurs because the light-sensing cells in the eye have been saturated with light from the laser. Any darkness usually resolves within a few hours. Rarely, the vision may become permanently blurred.

Visudyne is a photo-sensitizing drug that makes all tissues in the body very sensitive to light for about two days. For this reason, you must avoid any exposure to sunlight for two days after treatment; otherwise, severe skin burns may occur. Your doctor may advise you to wear long sleeves and a hat to his or her office, to prevent burns from sun exposure after your treatment.

Other side effects of photodynamic therapy include transient headache, back pain, and possible blurred or reduced vision.

Thermal Laser Therapy

Thermal laser therapy, also called *laser photo-coagulation,* is an FDA-approved treatment for wet macular degeneration that heats and destroys the abnormal blood vessels under the retina. The downside of this therapy is that it also damages the retina and causes an immediate and permanent blind spot in the area of vision. If this blind spot is located in the central macula, then there is loss of central vision. Typically, however, this vision loss is less than the amount of vision loss that would have eventually occurred without treatment.

With thermal laser therapy, it is likely that abnormal blood vessel growth will recur and the procedure will need to be repeated. Because of the immediate loss of vision that accompanies thermal laser therapy, it is rarely used for the treatment of wet macular degeneration.

Treatment for End-Stage Macular Degeneration

Most treatments for macular degeneration are designed to prevent the disease from reaching the end stage. End-stage macular degeneration occurs when the dry form develops into the wet form and then progresses to a point that is so severe that visual impairment is profound. Unfortunately, in some people, the disease will progress to the end stage, which is called disciform macular degeneration.

In disciform macular degeneration, development of scar tissue in the macular region permanently damages the central vision. There is little in the way of treatment for this condition. The management is aimed at utilizing the unaffected part of the macula to maximize a patient's remaining vision. This is done by way of low-vision aids and, more recently in some selected cases, with Implantable Miniature Telescopes (IMTs).

Implantable Miniature Telescope

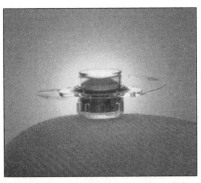

In 2010, the Implantable Miniature Telescope was approved by the FDA for use in those who have end-stage macular degeneration. The device is used to improve central vision. *Photo courtesy of VisonCare Opthalmic Technologies.*

The Implantable Miniature Telescope, approved by the FDA in 2010, is designed for use in individuals who have end-stage macular degeneration in both eyes. This tiny device, which is approximately the size of a pea, magnifies images so that they can be projected onto healthier portions of the retina, outside of the central area that has been damaged by macular degeneration.

The device is implanted in only one eye, allowing that eye to provide central vision while the eye without the device provides peripheral vision. Most people with the telescope implant experience significant improvement in vision. With the device implanted, some people may be able to regain the ability to recognize faces or facial expressions.

Not everyone with end-stage macular degeneration is a candidate for the telescope implant. You may be a candidate if you meet all of the following criteria:

- You have irreversible, end-stage macular degeneration resulting from either dry or wet macular degeneration.
- You are no longer a candidate for drug treatment of your macular degeneration.

- You have not had cataract surgery in the eye in which the telescope will be implanted.
- You meet age, vision, and cornea health requirements.

Before having surgery to implant the telescope, you will be asked to work with a *low-vision specialist,* using an external telescope, to see if you are likely to benefit from the telescope implant. Testing your vision with the external telescope will give you an idea of what your vision could be like with the telescope implant. Use of the telescope implant takes considerable training, but if your vision improves with an external telescope, you may be a candidate for the IMT.

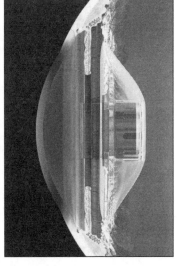

How the Telescope Is Implanted

Implantation of this device is a surgical procedure that is typically performed on an outpatient basis by a specially trained ophthalmic surgeon. You will be awake during the procedure, but

Implantable Miniature Telescope replaces the natural lens and is surgically inserted in only one eye. *Photo courtesy of Vison-Care Opthalmic Technologies.*

your eye will be numbed to minimize any discomfort during the procedure. Eyedrops will be administered to temporarily enlarge your pupil. During the procedure, your eye's natural lens will be removed, and the telescope will be inserted in its place.

In some cases, the eye surgeon may determine

during surgery that the eye is not compatible with the telescope implant. When this occurs, a standard intraocular lens will be implanted instead. An intraocular lens is the type of lens that is implanted during cataract surgery. The lens will not have any effect—positive or negative—on the visual impairment associated with macular degeneration.

After the Implant Procedure

After you have surgery for implantation of the device, you will need to participate in several training sessions with a low-vision specialist. The specialist will help you adapt to the way the telescope implant changes your vision. By working with your low-vision specialist, and practicing on your own at home, you can gain confidence in performing your daily activities with your new device.

Side Effects of the Telescope Implant

The most common side effects of the implant include increased eye pressure and inflammatory deposits on the device. Significant adverse effects include corneal swelling, the need for corneal transplant, and decrease in visual acuity.

In Summary

- The goal of treatment for macular degeneration is to delay the progress of the disease, prevent further vision loss, and, if possible, improve vision.
- Taking supplements of antioxidant micronutrients has been found to be helpful in the

management of dry macular degeneration.

- Major advances in the treatment of wet macular degeneration have been made in recent years.
- The treatment of choice for wet macular degeneration is one or two monthly injections of drugs called anti-VEGF and VEGF-Trap agents. Lucentis and Avastin have been the most frequently used anti-VEGF drugs. A newer VEGF-Trap drug called Eylea was approved by the FDA for wet macular degeneration in November 2011.
- Anti-VEGF and VEGF-Trap drugs stabilize the condition in over 90 percent of patients. These drugs result in visual improvement in about one-third of patients.
- When used for the treatment of wet macular degeneration, the benefits of anti-VEGF and VEGF-Trap drugs far outweigh their potential risks and side effects.
- In some cases of wet macular degeneration, a treatment called photodynamic therapy is used in combination with anti-VEGF drug injections.
- An older treatment called thermal laser therapy is rarely used today.
- Certain people with end-stage macular degeneration may benefit from an Implantable Miniature Telescope.

You may find it comforting to know that modern advances have made treatment for macular degeneration more effective than ever.

5 Reducing the Risk of Macular Degeneration Progression

When you have macular degeneration, one of the main goals of treatment is to reduce the risk that the condition will progress. Important ways to do this include regularly monitoring your eye health and improving your overall physical health. Did you know that eye health is correlated with general health? Taking care of your overall health is helpful in reducing the risk of macular degeneration progressing.

The Importance of Routine Eye Examinations

One of the most important steps you can take to reduce the risk of further vision loss is to monitor your condition on a regular basis. This includes scheduling eye examinations with your eye care professional as recommended. It also involves using self-testing tools, such as the Amsler grid, on a daily basis. Self-monitoring is very important because early detection is key to preventing any further deterioration of vision. If you notice any changes in your vision—including any new or increased distortion, blurring, or blank spots—report them as soon as possible to your eye care professional. Do *not* wait for your regularly scheduled exam. Delaying care may lead to permanent vision damage.

Reducing the Risk of Cardiovascular Disease

Having risk factors for cardiovascular disease, including high blood pressure, abnormal cholesterol levels, and smoking, increases the likelihood that macular degeneration will progress. Controlling these risk factors can be helpful in slowing the progression of macular degeneration.

Control Blood Pressure

High blood pressure is a condition in which the force of blood pushing against the walls of the arteries rises—and stays—above normal. High blood pressure is also referred to as hypertension. It is a known risk factor for heart disease and stroke. It has also been linked with an increased risk for wet macular degeneration.

Fortunately, there are many ways to control blood pressure. Many people are able to reduce high blood pressure with simple lifestyle interventions, such as reducing the amount of salt in the diet, getting regular exercise, and maintaining a healthy weight. When lifestyle interventions are not enough, your doctor may prescribe medication to control your blood pressure.

Control Cholesterol Levels

Cholesterol is a waxy, fatlike substance that circulates in the bloodstream. Cholesterol is essential to good health and helps the body make hormones, vitamin D, and many other important substances. However, cholesterol levels outside the normal range are associated with a higher incidence of heart attack and stroke as well as an increased risk for macular degeneration. Because of this, it is important to control cholesterol levels by eating a healthy diet, engaging in regular physical activity, and managing your weight. When these lifestyle changes are not enough, your physician may prescribe medication to help control your cholesterol levels.

Quit Smoking

Quitting smoking can decrease your risk of developing cardiovascular disease. It is also an important action you can take to reduce your risk of developing macular degeneration and slow the progression of the disease. Research shows that smoking leads to oxidative damage in the macula and also interferes with the absorption of lutein, a micronutrient that protects retinal cells from damage. Having low levels of lutein has been associated with a higher risk for advanced macular degeneration.

Stopping smoking is very challenging. The desire to prevent further vision loss from macular degeneration may provide added motivation to quit. Many programs and products are available to help you quit smoking, including nicotine patches, behavior modification programs, and even hypnosis. It may take several attempts to quit before you are successful, but the benefits of quitting are well worth it.

Exercise Regularly

Most people are aware that getting regular exercise decreases the risk of developing cardiovascular disease. But did you know that it also reduces the likelihood of developing wet macular degeneration? In one study, people who exercised at least three times a week were 70 percent less likely to develop wet macular degeneration than sedentary people.

Getting regular exercise does not mean you have to run marathons or join an expensive gym. Dancing, playing golf, or simply walking briskly for thirty minutes at least three times a week can provide health benefits. You can likely find many opportunities to engage in physical activity in your community.

Nutrition for Optimal Eye Health

While the role of diet in preventing the progression of macular degeneration is still being investigated, there is ample evidence that eating a nutritious diet can improve your eye health as well as your overall physical well-being. Because of this, adopting sound dietary practices is highly encouraged.

Eat Fruits and Vegetables

A growing body of research has found that consuming antioxidant-rich, disease-fighting fruits and vegetables may help prevent macular degeneration and its progression. In particular, scientists have found that eating fruits and vegetables that are high in the antioxidant pigment nutrients called lutein and *zeaxanthin* may offer some protection from macular degeneration. This protection may be related to the fact that lutein and zeaxanthin are found in high concentrations in the macula. When levels of these substances are low, there may be a higher risk that macular degeneration will develop.

Fruits and vegetables that are high in lutein and zeaxanthin include:

- broccoli
- brussels sprouts
- collard greens
- corn
- kale
- kiwi
- orange bell peppers
- oranges
- red grapes
- romaine lettuce
- spinach
- turnip greens
- zucchini

Choose Fats Wisely

Fat has gotten a bad reputation, but it's important to realize that not all fats are created equal. Yes, there are some "bad" fats that are best to avoid. But there are also "good" fats that promote good health, including good eye health.

Fats that may be harmful to health include the following:

- *Saturated fats:* Found mainly in animal fat, these fats raise low-density lipoprotein (LDL), or "bad," cholesterol levels.
- *Trans fats:* These fats—which raise LDL cholesterol levels and lower high-density lipoprotein (HDL), or "good," cholesterol levels—are typically found in processed foods, including store-bought crackers, cookies, and chips.

Fats that may contribute to good health include the following:

- *Monounsaturated fats:* Found in a variety of foods and oils, such as avocados and olive oil, these fats promote healthy cholesterol levels and decrease the risk of cardiovascular disease.
- *Polyunsaturated fats:* These fats, which are found in plant-based foods and oils, improve cholesterol levels. Omega-3 fatty acids, which are a particular type of polyunsaturated fat, may offer protection against macular degeneration. One study found that people who consumed the highest amounts of omega-3 fatty acids had a 30 percent lower risk of developing macular degeneration than those who consumed the lowest amounts. Omega-3 fatty acids are found in:
  - flaxseed oil
  - flaxseeds
  - herring
  - salmon
  - sardines
  - tuna
  - walnuts

Choose the Right Carbohydrates

Choosing the right carbohydrates is also key. Focus on whole-grain carbohydrates, which are high in fiber. Foods that are high in fiber help lower blood pressure and control cholesterol. Plus, they make you feel full longer, so they can be helpful when you are trying to lose weight.

Start with Small Changes

Many people find it easier to start with a few lifestyle adjustments rather than attempt to make drastic changes all at once. Adopting a few new healthy behaviors can have a big impact on your overall health, which may help prevent further vision loss.

In Summary

- Reducing the risk of the disease progressing is one of the main goals of treatment for macular degeneration.
- Seeing your eye care specialist for routine eye exams is one of the most important things you can do to reduce the risk of further vision loss.
- To reduce the risk of the disease progressing, lower your risk factors for cardiovascular disease, quit smoking, and exercise on a regular basis.
- Eat a healthy diet that includes fruits and vegetables, good fats, and high-fiber whole grains.
- Making just a few small lifestyle changes can have a big impact on your health, including your eye health.

Making smart lifestyle choices on a daily basis can play a major role in reducing your risk of further vision loss due to macular degeneration.

6 Living with Macular Degeneration

As you likely already know, living with macular degeneration requires making some adjustments. Fortunately, a vast array of resources are available that can help you adapt so that you can continue living a full life. Your eye care professional can point you to other specialists who can assist you and to tools that may aid you. There are also several simple strategies you can employ to help you deal with the changes in your vision.

It is important to remember that your ability to adapt relies not only on external assistance but also, in large part, on your own "can do" attitude. A willingness to change and try new strategies can make a big difference in your ability to thrive. It is also important to recognize that although macular degeneration can severely diminish your central vision for reading and driving, it rarely affects your peripheral vision. Most people with macular degeneration retain good enough vision to be able to perform most of their daily tasks.

Low-Vision Specialists

If you are experiencing any bothersome vision loss due to macular degeneration, your retinal specialist may refer you to a low-vision specialist. These specialists are licensed doctors of optometry or oph-thalmology who are trained in helping people manage the challenges of low vision.

Although low-vision specialists are not able to restore the vision you have lost, they will introduce you to tools and techniques that can enhance your daily life, and they will train you to use the tools and use the vision you have more effectively. They will take into account your current lifestyle, career, and hobbies in order to find the best resources for you.

It is important to remember that low-vision devices take some time and effort to learn to use them effectively. Some specialists will also schedule home visits, to recommend ways to make your home more "eye-friendly."

Low-Vision Support Aids

Many tools and gadgets have been developed to help people with visual impairment resulting from macular degeneration. Popular low-vision support aids include:

- magnifiers
- eyeglass filters
- computers
- reading machines
- phones
- clocks, watches, and calculators
- lamps and other lighting
- voice-activated notetakers

Magnifiers

Magnifiers are some of the most useful devices for people with visual impairment due to macular degeneration. They come in a wide variety of models.

Handheld magnifiers: Commonly known as magnifying glasses, these handy tools come in a range of sizes and are capable of magnifying objects up to five times the actual size. Some handheld magnifiers come equipped with battery-operated lighting. Many are small enough to slip into a pocket or handbag, so you can take them with you when shopping, dining out, or doing similar activities. The advantages of

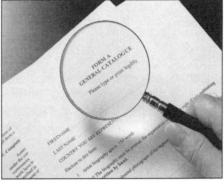

Handheld magnifying glasses are portable and economical.

handheld magnifiers are low cost and portability. The disadvantages include relatively limited field of vision and relatively lower magnification. They also can be difficult to use if you suffer from hand tremors.

Stand magnifiers: Larger than handheld magnifiers, these magnifiers are mounted on stands that can be placed on any flat surface; they are available in both desktop and floor lamp styles. These devices are helpful for reading, writing, and similar tasks.

Stand magnifiers usually come with a light source. Available in electric and battery-operated versions, lighted stand magnifiers are called magnifying lamps. Magnifying lamps are also commonly used by den-

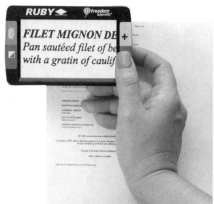

Handheld video magnifiers can be used for reading small print, product labels, medicine bottle labels, menus, or appliance controls. *Photo courtesy of Freedom Scientific.*

tists, watch repairers, and other professionals who specialize in fine-detail work. What does a magnifying lamp look like? Think of a typical desktop lamp or floor lamp that has an adjustable arm. Now envision that the light source is in the shape of a circle or rectangle surrounding a magnifying lens. You simply position the illuminated magnifier over a book or close-up task for easier viewing.

Stand magnifiers are available at many office supply stores or from online low-vision specialty retailers. The advantages of stand magnifiers are steadiness and higher magnification. The disadvantages include higher cost and less portability.

Eyeglass-mounted magnifiers: Small magnifiers can be attached to eyeglasses to provide assistance with either distance or up-close vision. Tiny telescopes help with distance vision; microscopes improve near vision. These eyeglass-mounted magnifiers are typically available by prescription from low-vision specialists.

Binoculars: Specialized low-vision binoculars come in models that magnify either distance or near vision in both eyes. Distance-vision enhancers are good for viewing sporting events, watching TV, or

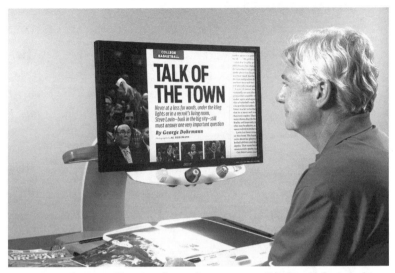

Video magnifiers provide crisp, clear enlargements and help you do such things as read small print, sign checks, or write letters. *Photo courtesy of Freedom Scientific.*

watching movies at the cinema. Models designed for near vision help with close-up tasks. Most models allow you to adjust each eye separately for maximum clarity.

Monoculars: These distance-vision tools are similar to binoculars, but are designed for one eye only.

Video magnifiers: These devices, also known as closed-circuit televisions (CCTVs), feature a video camera mounted on a stand. You simply point the video camera at the object you want to magnify, and the enlarged image appears on a video screen. These aids are very useful for reading, writing, and doing crafts. The downsides of video magnifiers include high cost and reduced field of vision.

Eyeglass Filters

Specialized eyeglass filters known as absorptive filters increase contrast, reduce glare, and ease the transition between light and dark environments. These filters are available in a variety of colors, including amber and yellow, and some may be worn over your regular eyeglasses.

Computers

Computers can be modified for low vision with a number of helpful products. Large-print, high-contrast keyboards are easier to see, even in low light. Large monitors and screen magnifiers enlarge

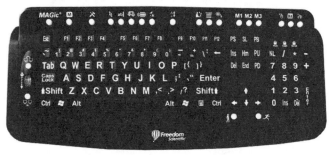

Large-print keyboards make it easier to work at a computer. *Photo courtesy of Freedom Scientific.*

the images you see on the screen. Voice recognition programs allow you to use voice commands with your computer. Screen-reading software programs that talk provide another useful tool to facilitate computer use.

If you use the Internet, note that many Web sites have adjustable font sizes and contrast for easier reading.

Reading Machines

Reading machines are devices that scan images of handwritten or printed text and read it back to you aloud. Available in desktop or portable models, reading machines can help you read books, newspapers, food labels, bills, and more. Specialized software, known as optical character recognition software, can also turn your computer into a reading machine.

Phones

Phones with large, lighted numbers can make it easier to place and receive calls. Some phones allow you to make calls, answer calls, and converse simply by using your voice. In some areas, visual loss from macular degeneration may qualify you for free directory assistance from your phone company.

Clocks, Watches, and Calculators

Wall clocks, alarm clocks, desk clocks, travel clocks, wristwatches, stopwatches, and timers designed specifically for people with low vision can help you tell time. These products talk, vibrate, or have large numbers. Similarly, calculators with large-number, high-contrast buttons and high-contrast displays offer enhanced visibility.

Lamps and Other Lighting

A wide range of lamps and other lighting devices are designed to provide bright light, increase contrast, and decrease glare. The light bulbs you use can also make a difference. Some people with macular degeneration prefer halogen light bulbs because they tend to produce less glare than incandescent or fluorescent light bulbs.

Voice-Activated Notetakers

Making a to-do list, taking notes in a meeting, or noting reminders to take medications is easier with voice-activated note-taking. Many handheld digital recorders offer this feature, and the devices are small enough to keep in a pocket or purse when not in use.

Calendars and Address Books

Large-print calendars and address books can be helpful. These typically have bold lines and type so they are easier to see.

Record-Keeping and Check-Writing Aids

To help you maintain your independence, there are a number of low-vision aids that facilitate record-keeping and check-writing. For example, signature guides are simple devices that help you sign your name in the appropriate place on checks, contracts, and other documents. You may also order raised-letter or large-print checks from the bank.

Strategies for Dealing with Vision Changes

A number of simple strategies can help you adapt to the visual changes associated with macular degeneration. By using these techniques, you can make your surroundings more comfortable, boost your confidence, and enhance your everyday life.

Improve Lighting

Consider positioning lights, magnifying lights, desk lamps, and light bulbs strategically throughout your home. Make sure you have good lighting in places where you spend a lot of time and where you tend to read or write. For safety purposes, use ample lighting in entryways, stairways, basements, and attics. Use nightlights in any room of the house you may walk through at night. This is preferable to switching on a bright light, because when you have macular degeneration, it typically takes longer to adjust to changes in light. To minimize glare, consider shutting curtains, blinds, shades, or shutters during the brightest times of the day.

Increase Contrast

Increasing the contrast between light and dark objects in your home can help you navigate your way around and locate things. For example, place dark-colored furniture in front of light walls, or a light-colored lamp next to a dark chair. Having furniture, tables, walls, and window dressings all in a neutral color palette can make it difficult to distinguish items. Similarly, busy patterns on furniture, window dressings, or walls can make it harder to judge where things are.

For the best effect, increase contrast in every room of the house, including the bathroom, kitchen, and dining room. For example, in the bathroom, you may want to consider getting a dark lid for a light toilet. Put lotions, gels, and other personal hygiene products in containers with colors that contrast with the sink top. In the kitchen, use dark or light pots and pans to contrast with the stove. For dining, choose tablecloths in shades that contrast with your dinnerware. Use light cups for dark liquids, and dark containers to store light-colored liquids, such as milk. This enables you to better judge fluid levels.

Get Organized

Keeping your household organized is essential. Eliminate clutter around the house to prevent tripping or falling. Organize your bills, keys, reading material, jewelry, and other items into clearly labeled bins or baskets to prevent things from getting lost or misplaced. This can greatly reduce frustration and enhance your quality of life.

Establish Consistency and Routine

Consistency and routine can be important coping strategies for dealing with macular degeneration. Keeping everything in the same place on countertops, in drawers, and in cupboards simplifies everyday activities, such as bathing, getting dressed, and preparing food. Enlist the support of your family and guests in this endeavor, and ask them not to move items from their usual places.

Practice Using Your Side Vision

Because macular degeneration does not affect your side vision (also called peripheral vision), it is a good idea to practice using this vision. Try tilting your head up or down or turning it to the side to find your best vision, and practice looking at things that way. This may take some getting used to, so start with just a few minutes at a time and gradually increase the length of time you focus using your noncentral vision.

Sharpen Your Other Senses

In the rare case that vision becomes significantly impaired, it is a good idea to sharpen your other senses so you can learn to utilize them more effectively. People with end-stage macular degeneration may devise systems using touch to help differentiate objects. For example, you might use rubber bands to identify jars of food—one rubber band for green beans, two rubber bands for corn, and so on. When pouring liquids into a glass or cup, you may want to hold the glass or cup in such a way that your thumb will feel when the liquid reaches a certain level.

Tune in to your sense of hearing. Sharpening your listening skills may take some adjustment at first but can prove to be very beneficial. For example, hearing a "talking" clock may signal that you are nearing your bedside, or hearing the hum of the refrigerator may indicate that you are entering the kitchen.

Coping in the Workplace

It is important to come up with a coping strategy for the workplace. An important first step may be to speak with your employer about accommodations that can be made to help you perform your job to the best of your ability. Part of being independent is knowing when to ask for help.

Apply the same strategies as at home—improving lighting, increasing contrast, getting organized, establishing consistency and routine, and sharpening your other senses—to your office and work activities to enhance your productivity. Today more than ever before, it is possible for people with macular degeneration to maintain active and productive careers.

Enjoying Travel and Recreation

Each and every day, tens of thousands of people with macular degeneration enjoy traveling and engaging in their favorite recreational activities. Depending on your level of vision loss, you may benefit from advance planning, specialized tools, or assistance. Here are some tips to help you get the most out of your leisure pursuits.

Travel

Whether you want to explore your local neighborhood, enjoy a relaxing cruise vacation, or journey to a far-off, exotic locale, special assistance may be available. For example, a number of travel agencies specialize in booking trips for people with disabilities, including low vision. Directories of these agencies are available online. Many airlines, cruise lines, train stations, and hotels also offer information and assistance to make travel easier for people with visual impairment, and some even provide discounts. Check their Web sites for more information.

When traveling, follow these suggestions:

- Always arrive early at the airport, train station, bus terminal, or cruise ship to allow extra time for navigating the area.

- Notify customer service representatives or travel personnel that you are visually impaired, and if needed, ask for an escort to your departure or baggage claim area.
- Preboard to give yourself more time to find your seat and stow any carry-on bags.
- Use bright, colorful tags to identify your luggage, or consider buying luggage in a bright color.
- When visiting tourist attractions, consider renting the audio tour of the facility, which may be free to people with visual impairment.

Recreation

Thanks to specialized products, having macular degeneration doesn't mean you have to give up your favorite games, crafts, hobbies, or other recreational activities.

Games: Large-print playing cards and board games are widely available. So are large-print books of popular word games and puzzles. A growing number of video games for the visually impaired use sound cues instead of images.

Crafts: Self-threading needles can enable you to enjoy hobbies such as needlepoint and cross-stitching. Knitters can take advantage of knitting patterns available in large-print type and speech formats. Crafts that rely more heavily on the sense of touch, including sculpting and ceramics, may be good options to try.

Gardening: If you love to garden, there is no reason why macular degeneration should keep you from engaging in this activity. Here are a few suggestions to make this hobby safer and more enjoyable for you:

- Because wet grass, slippery rocks, and uneven ground levels pose tripping hazards, it is wise to make a few simple changes to help keep yourself safe. Create a walkway using nonslippery surfaces, and make sure it is even.
- Choose gardening tools with brightly colored handles, and devise a system to identify the tools.
- Choose plants in bright colors.

Books, Magazines, Newspapers, and Movies: For people with end-stage macular degeneration, listening to books, magazines, and newspapers on tape or CD can be an enjoyable alternative to reading. Many cinemas and home DVDs offer Descriptive Video Service (DVS) for the visually impaired. With this feature, you can hear descriptions of the visual details of a film to enhance the viewing experience.

Adapting to Social Situations

If your vision loss is severe, you may need to adapt in social situations. In our society, it is common to look someone in the eye when meeting or saying hello. But when you have end-stage macular degeneration with significant loss of central vision, it is likely that your best vision is your peripheral, or side, vision. For this reason, you may find that you need to move your eyes up, down, or to the side to get the best view of people's faces. You may want to let people know that you have macular degeneration and briefly explain how it affects your vision, so they will understand why you aren't looking at them directly.

Engaging Family and Friends

Getting your family and friends on board with your coping strategies can be helpful. As noted earlier, be sure to inform them that it is important to refrain from moving items from their usual places in your home.

As you go about your daily routine, you may find that family, friends, and even strangers want to help you spontaneously with things such as opening a door, getting up from a couch, or finding an elevator button. Depending on your level of vision loss, you may want to respond by saying something such as, "Thank you, but I'm fine in handling this situation. Don't worry about me." Or, if you do need help, speak up. For example, you might say, "I could use help with these steps, please."

Finding Outside Support

Joining a support group may have a positive impact on your life. Support groups can have great healing power emotionally. Perhaps most importantly, these groups take you out of your isolation and put you in touch with others who are taking the same journey as you. There is great comfort in this—you don't feel so alone with your situation. That, in itself, is powerful.

Support groups offer you the chance to openly share your feelings about your vision loss and any changes it has caused in your life. On the practical side, meeting with other people who have macular degeneration also gives you the opportunity to swap strategies on how to cope with daily living. For these reasons, many people find joining a support group to be a very rewarding experience.

A final point about support groups: If, at first, you don't think the meetings are right for you, be patient. Psychologists recommend that you attend at least five or six such meetings before you decide whether a support group is right for you.

Regular Retinal Evaluations

When you develop wet macular degeneration, regular eye examinations and treatments become an important part of your life routine. Although this may seem inconvenient, regular retinal evaluations can save your sight. These evaluations are usually done every one to two months. Once the condition stabilizes, the interval between evaluations may be increased gradually. You should allow up to three hours for each retinal evaluation in order to have all the necessary examinations, tests, and possible treatments done during the same visit.

It is prudent to monitor your own vision on a daily basis in between evaluations by your retinal specialist. You can do this by using the Amsler grid or a similar visual grid, such as a door frame or computer graphics.

In Summary

- Your retinal specialist may refer you to a low-vision specialist, who can point you to products that can enhance your life.
- A vast array of low-vision tools can help you live with macular degeneration.
- A number of simple strategies can help you adapt to the visual changes associated with macular degeneration.
- Coping strategies can be helpful at home, in the workplace, while traveling, or while engaging in your favorite leisure activities.
- Engaging the support of friends and family or joining a support group may have a positive impact on your life.

A growing variety of readily available tools and coping strategies make it easier to live with the challenges of vision loss due to macular degeneration.

Appendix

Amsler Grid

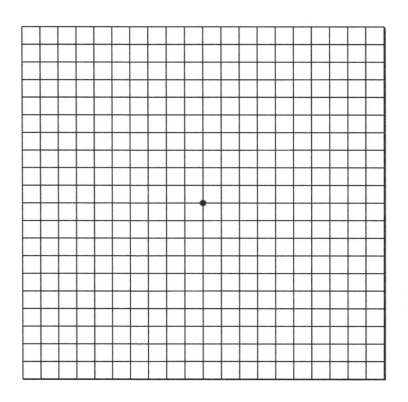

Resources

AMD Alliance International
6th Floor, City Gate East, Tollhouse Hill
Nottingham, NG1 5SF
United Kingdom
Phone: (44) 115-935-2100

10519 Old Court Road
Woodstock, MD 21163
www.amdalliance.org

American Academy of Ophthalmology
P.O. Box 7424
San Francisco, CA 94120-7424
Phone: (415) 561-8500
www.aao.org

American Macular Degeneration Foundation
P.O. Box 515
Northampton, MA 01061-0515
Phone: (888) MACULAR (622-8527)
www.macular.org

American Optometric Association
243 North Lindbergh Boulevard
St. Louis, MO 63141
Phone: (800) 365-2219
www.aoa.org

American Society of Retina Specialists
20 North Wacker Drive, Suite 2234
Chicago, IL 60606
Phone: (312) 578-8760
www.asrs.org

Association for Macular Diseases, Inc.
210 East 64th Street
New York, NY 10065
Phone: (212) 605-3719
www.macula.org

The Macula Foundation
210 East 64th Street
New York, NY 10065
Phone: (800) 622-8524 / (212) 605-3777
www.maculafoundation.org

Macular Degeneration Association
P.O. Box 20256
Sarasota, FL 34276
Phone: (941) 870-4399
www.maculardegenerationassociation.org

Macular Degeneration Foundation
P.O. Box 531313
Henderson, NV 89053
Phone: (888) 633-3937 / (702) 450-2908
www.eyesight.org

Macular Degeneration Partnership
6222 Wilshire Boulevard, Suite 260
Los Angeles, CA 90048
Phone: (310) 623-4466
www.amd.org

Macular Degeneration Research: A Program of the American Health Assistance Foundation
22512 Gateway Center Drive
Clarksburg, MD 20871
Phone: (800) 437-2423
www.ahaf.org/macular

MD Support
3600 Blue Ridge Boulevard
Grandview, MO 64030
Phone: (816) 761-7080
www.mdsupport.org

National Eye Institute/ National Institutes of Health
2020 Vision Place
Bethesda, MD 20892-3655
Phone: (301) 496-5248
www.nei.nih.gov

L.A. Retina Vitreous Associates
8641 Wilshire Blvd., Ste. 210
Beverly Hills, CA 90211
Phone: (310) 854-6201
www.laretina.com
www.maculainfo.org
www.retinainfor.org

Glossary

A

Age-Related Eye Disease Study (AREDS): A study that found that taking high doses of certain vitamins and minerals reduced the risk of developing advanced macular degeneration.

Age-related macular degeneration (AMD): A degenerative condition that affects the center portion of the retina known as the macula. Also called macular degeneration.

Amblyopia: An imbalance between a person's eyes during early childhood that leads to permanent loss of vision. Also called "lazy eye."

Amsler grid: A grid with a dark dot in the center, used to test for visual symptoms such as distortion of vision that may signify the onset of wet macular degeneration.

Angiography: A process of obtaining images of blood vessels within and under the retina that retinal surgeons use to determine how best to stop the vessels from leaking.

Anterior chamber: The fluid-filled space inside the eye behind the cornea and in front of the iris.

Antioxidant: An agent that reduces the damage due to by-products of the normal chemical reactions with oxygen in the body.

Anti-VEGF (vascular endothelial growth factor) drug: A drug that targets abnormal blood vessel growth.

Arteriosclerosis: Thickening of the walls of the arteries.

Artery: A blood vessel that carries oxygenated blood to the tissues of the body.

Atherosclerosis: The accumulation of fatty deposits on the walls of large blood vessels.

B

Beta-carotene: A type of vitamin called a carotenoid. Related to vitamin A.

Blank spots: A commonly reported symptom of macular degeneration in which areas of the patient's view disappear.

Blotches: A commonly reported symptom of macular degeneration in which gray or black stains appear in the patient's view.

Blue light: A portion of the light spectrum that is suspected of being harmful to the retina.

Blurring: A commonly reported symptom of macular degeneration in which lines or edges of objects in the patient's view lose their sharpness.

Bruch's membrane: The thin, compact membrane located between the retina and the underlying flat carpet of blood vessels that supply the retina with nourishment.

C

Carotenoid: Any of the yellow to red pigments found widely in plants and foods such as carrots or red tomatoes.

Cataract: A clouding of the lens of the eye that causes decreased vision.

Central atrophy: A thinning of the retina that occurs as part of macular degeneration.

Central serous retinopathy: A malfunction of the retinal pigment epithelium that allows fluid to leak under the retina, causing a limited retinal detachment.

Central vision: Vision used for reading and fine-detail work.

Cholesterol: A waxy substance that can accumulate on the walls of arteries and cause health problems.

Choroid: The network of blood vessels under the retina. The choroid provides blood supply to the overlying retina photoreceptors.

Choroidal neovascularization (CNV): A process in which abnormal blood vessels grow from the small blood vessels in the choroid under the retina. CNV is most commonly caused by wet macular degeneration.

Classic wet macular degeneration: A type of wet macular degeneration characterized by rapid leaking of fluids under the retina and rapidly appearing visual problems.

Closed-circuit television (CCTV): A technology that uses a video camera to place objects on a screen at increased magnification.

Cold laser: A low-intensity laser that does not produce heat. It is commonly used in conjunction with Visudyne infusion for photodynamic treatment of some forms of wet macular degeneration.

Comparison of Age-Related Macular Degeneration Treatment Trial (CATT): A study that found that the drugs Lucentis and Avastin are equally effective for the treatment of wet macular degeneration.

Conjunctiva: The mucous membrane that lines the inside of the eyelids and extends over the front of the white part of the eye.

Cornea: The transparent outermost part of the eye that helps focus the image.

D

Diagnose: To determine the cause of an illness or medical condition.

Dilate: To enlarge, as the pupils.

Disability: An impairment that affects a person's ability to perform certain daily functions.

Disciform scarring: Severe and irreversible scarring of the macula that is associated with end-stage macular degeneration.

Distortion: A commonly reported symptom of macular degeneration in which lines in the patient's view appear wavy.

Dominant eye: The eye that works harder than the other.

Drusen: Small, yellow mounds of debris that accumulate within Bruch's membrane and are often an early sign of macular degeneration.

Dry eye: A condition that occurs when the tear film loses its ability to adequately lubricate the eye.

Dry macular degeneration: A condition associated with a gradual breakdown of cells in the macula.

E

Enzyme: A special protein that acts as a promoter during chemical reactions in the body.

Exudate: A clear fluid.

F

Floater: Seen as a spot, a particle that floats in the vitreous and creates a shadow on the retina.

Fluorescein: A special dye used for visualizing blood vessels under the retina.

Fovea: The center part of the macula that provides the sharpest vision.

Free radical: An unstable, high-energy molecule. Free radicals are toxic substances produced by all cells in the body.

Fundus fluorescein angiography: A technique used for visualizing blood vessels under the retina.

G

Geographic atrophy: A condition in which the loss of retinal photoreceptors, retinal pigment epithelial cells, and choroidal vessels occurs around the macula in a patchy pattern.

Glaucoma: A disorder of the eye characterized by an increase of pressure within the eyeball.

H

HDL (high-density lipoprotein) cholesterol: The "good" form of cholesterol that removes cholesterol from the body.

High blood pressure: Abnormal elevation of the pressure of blood in the arteries produced by the pumping action of the heart. Also called hypertension.

Hypertension: *See* High blood pressure.

I

Idiopathic: Refering to disease of unknown origin or without apparent cause.

Indirect ophthalmoscopy: A diagnostic test utilizing a special headset light and handheld magnifier that allows visualization of the peripheral retina and an overview of the macula and nerve of the eye.

Infection: An inflammation in body tissue caused by microorganisms.

Inflammation: A natural response in the body to fight disease and infection that, when it becomes chronic, is associated with increased risk for further disease.

Intraocular lens: A type of lens implanted during cataract surgery.

Intraocular pressure: Pressure within the eye.

Iris: The tissue in front of the lens that opens and closes to control the amount of light entering the eye. The iris is the structure that gives color to the eye.

L

Laser photocoagulation: An outdated treatment for wet macular degeneration that involved the use of a laser to destroy leaky and abnormal blood vessels under the retina. Also called thermal laser therapy.

LDL (low-density lipoprotein) cholesterol: The "bad" form of cholesterol that is more likely to form the plaque that can block arteries.

Lens: The clear structure near the front of the eye that focuses images onto the retina. It has the same shape and function as the lens within a camera.

Lipid: Any of the fats in the body, including cholesterol.

Lipoprotein: A type of molecule consisting of fat and protein that carries cholesterol through the bloodstream.

Low vision: Reduced vision that cannot be corrected with eyeglasses or contact lenses.

Lutein: A micronutrient that protects retinal cells from damage.

M

Macula: The center of the retina, used for direct focusing.

Macular atrophy: Thinning of the macula.

Macular degeneration: The most common cause of legal blindness among people over age fifty. It involves degenerative changes in the central portion of the retina called the macula. It may lead to loss of central vision. Also called age-related macular degeneration.

Macular dystrophy: An abnormality in the cells of the retina due to gene defects that can cause symptoms of macular degeneration at an early age.

Macular hole: A microscopic hole that can appear in the macula.

Macular pucker: A layer of scar tissue on the eye's macula that causes blurred and distorted vision.

Macular translocation: A surgical procedure that relocates the macula away from leaking blood vessels. Macular translocation is rarely performed today.

Microscope: An instrument that provides magnified images of very tiny objects.

Monounsaturated fat: Any of a class of oils (including olive oil and canola oil) that are better for the body than saturated or polyunsaturated fats.

N

Neovascularization: The formation of new abnormal blood vessels, usually under or in the retina in wet macular degeneration.

Nerve: Any of the fibers containing nerve cells that convey impulses from the central nervous system to other parts of the body.

Neurologic: Referring to the nervous system.

O

Occult wet macular degeneration: A type of wet macular degeneration characterized by slower leakage of fluids under the retina.

Ophthalmologist: A medical doctor who specializes in the diagnosis, medical treatment, and surgical treatment of eye diseases.

Ophthalmoscope: A device used to shine a bright light into the eye.

Ophthalmoscopy: A diagnostic test used to examine the structures at the back of the eye.

Optical coherence tomography (OCT): A diagnostic test that uses light technology to produce a high-resolution scan of the macula.

Optic nerve: A nerve that transmits electrical impulses from the eye to the brain.

Optometrist: A licensed eye care professional who specializes in performing eye exams, prescribing lenses, and providing certain medical treatments.

Oxidation: A process in which certain by-products of oxygen use react with nearby molecules. In the body, oxidation is thought to cause damage to tissues.

P

Peripheral retina: The side areas of the retina.

Peripheral vision: Side vision.

Photodynamic therapy: The use of cold laser beams to activate special dyes in order to stop retinal bleeding.

Photoreceptor: A retinal cell that detects light. These cells enable us to see.

Photo-sensitizing dye: A dye that responds to light.

Pigment epithelial detachment (PED): A split occurring in Bruch's membrane that fills with fluid and causes a dome-shaped detachment of the pigment epithelium underlying the retina, leading to visual distortion or other symptoms. Pigment epithelial detachments are often associated with macular degeneration.

Pigment epithelium rip: A condition caused by a tear in the retinal pigment epithelium, leading to sudden loss of vision. Pigment epithelial rips are often associated with macular degeneration but can also result from direct trauma to the eye.

Polypoidal choroidal vasculopathy: Small swellings within the walls of blood vessels under the retina that burst and cause damage to the retina. In many instances, polypoidal choroidal vasculopathy is considered a variation of wet macular degeneration.

Polyunsaturated fat: A type of fat that helps rid the body of cholesterol but that should still be limited in a person's diet.

Pupil: The black circular part of the eye in the center of the iris that changes in size to regulate the amount of light entering the eye.

R

Receptor: Any of the cells that initiate and conduct signals to the brain and provide various sensory inputs such as vision and hearing.

Remodeling: A process by which the blank spots noted by patients using the Amsler grid change positions.

Retina: The part of the eye that contains the rods and the cones. It receives the image from the lens and conveys visual information to the brain via the optic nerve. The retina functions much like the film in a camera or the chip in a video camera.

Retinal detachment: A separation of the retina from the retinal pigment epithelium that requires immediate medical attention.

Retinal fibrosis: Scarring in the retina.

Retinal pigment epithelium (RPE): A single layer of cells between the retina and the underlying choroidal blood vessels.

Retinal specialist: An ophthalmologist specializing in diseases of the retina, including macular degeneration.

Risk factor: A behavior or physical trait that increases a person's risk of getting a disease.

S

Saturated fat: A type of fat found in red meats, some dairy products, and some plants. High levels of these fats are known to be harmful to the body, and so intake should be limited.

Slit lamp: A modified microscope with a bright light, used for examining the eye.

Snellen chart: A chart that typically contains rows of letters and is used to test visual acuity.

Stem cell: A type of primitive cell that can transform into and generate other cells.

Subretinal blood: Blood that has pooled under the retina.

Subretinal fluid: Fluid that has pooled under the retina.

Symptom: A physical manifestation of a disease.

T

Tear film: A layer of fluid that bathes and lubricates the cornea.

Tonometry: A test used to measure eye pressure. It uses blue light.

Tono-Pen: A device used to measure eye pressure.

20/20 vision: Ideal visual acuity. The first number indicates the standard distance (20 feet) a person is from an eye chart while being tested. The second number indicates the person's ability to identify the smallest line on the eye chart from 20 feet away.

U

Ultraviolet (UV) light: The nonvisible portion of the light spectrum, with a wavelength shorter than violet light.

V

Vascular endothelial growth factor (VEGF): A type of protein that stimulates the growth of abnormal blood vessels.

Visual acuity test: A measure of the clarity of one's vision.

Visual field test: A test used to measure peripheral vision.

Vitreous: The clear, jellylike fluid in the central portion of the eye.

Vitreous hemorrhage: A hemorrhage within the vitreous of the eye.

W

Wet macular degeneration: A type of macular degeneration characterized by leakage and bleeding from abnormal blood vessels growing into the space under the retina. Without timely treatment, wet macular degeneration causes permanent loss of central vision.

Z

Zeaxanthin: A micronutrient that may help prevent macular degeneration.

Zinc: An antioxidant mineral that neutralizes free radicals and is important to the proper functioning of the body.

Index

A

address books, 86

advanced stage of macular degeneration, 46

age/aging, 5, 16

Age-Related Eye Disease Study (AREDS), 56, 103

age-related macular degeneration (AMD), 1, 103. *See also* Macular degeneration

amblyopia, 103

AMD. *See* age-related macular degeneration (AMD)

Amsler grid test, 27–29, 39, 97, 103

anatomy of eye, 7

angiography, fundus fluorescein, 44, 47

anterior chamber, 41, 103

anti-VEGF (vascular endothelial growth factor) drugs, 13, 58–59, 63, 65

antioxidants, 19, 103

AREDS. *See* Age-Related Eye Disease Study (AREDS)

arteriosclerosis, 17, 104

artery, 104

atherosclerosis, 104

Avastin (bevacizumab), 59–60

B

back of the eye, examination of, 42–43

bad fats, 76

beta carotene, 56, 104

binoculars, 82–83

blank spots, 04, 24

blind spot, 42

blood pressure, control of, 73

blotches, 24, 104

blue light, 19, 104

blurring, 24, 104

Bonnet, C., 14

Bruch's membrane, 3, 104

C

calculators, 85

calendars, 86

carbohydrates, choosing, 77

cardiovascular system

    blood pressure, control of, 73

    cholesterol levels, control of, 73–74

    disease, reduction of risk

of, 73–77
exercise, regular, 75
risk factors for macular
degeneration, 17–18
smoking, quitting, 74
carotenoid, 104
cataract, 20, 104
cataract surgery, 20–21
CATT. *See* Comparison of
Age-Related Macular De-
generation Treatment Trial
(CATT)
CCTVs. *See* Closed-circuit
televisions (CCTVs)
central atrophy, 104
central serous retinopathy,
104
central vision, 10, 104
Charles Bonnet syndrome,
14–15, 26
check-writing aids, 86
cholesterol, 73–74, 105
choroid, 2, 105
choroidal blood vessels, 3
choroidal capillaries, 46
choroidal neovascularization
(CNV), 11, 105
classic wet macular degeneration, 11, 105
clocks, 85
closed-circuit televisions
(CCTVs), 83, 105
CNV. *See* choroidal neovascularization (CNV)
cold laser, 64–65, 105
Comparison of Age-Related
Macular Degeneration

Treatment Trial (CATT),
60, 105
computers, 84
conjunctiva, 40, 63, 105
contrast, increased, 87–88
copper, 56
cornea, 2, 41, 105
crafts, 91

D
descriptive video service
(DVS), 92
development process of
macular degeneration, 4
diagnose, defined, 32, 105
diagnosis for macular degeneration, 32–53
emotionally coping with,
51–52
eye care specialist for,
31–34, 51
eye examination for, 34–50
dilation, 105
disability, 106
disciform scarring, 9, 13, 106
diseased retina, 34
distortion, 24, 106
dominant eye, 106
drug injections, 58–63
process for giving, 61–62
side effects of, 62–63
drusen, 5, 8, 106
dry eye, 41, 106
dry macular degeneration, 6
characteristics of, 6
defined, 6, 106
development of, 4
early symptoms of, 23–25

home monitoring for, 57
managing, 55–57
nutritional supplements
for, 55–57
optical coherence tomography of, 49
progression of, 25
severe cases of, 6
signs of, 43
vitamins for, 55–57
DVS. *See* descriptive video
service (DVS)

E
early detection of macular
degeneration, importance
of, 30
early stages of macular degeneration, 45–46
emotionally coping with diagnosis for macular degeneration, 51–52
end-stage macular degeneration, 67
enzyme, 106
ethnicity as risk factors for
macular degeneration, 16
exercise, regular, 75
existing macular degeneration
as risk factors for macular
degeneration, 20
exudate, 106
eye
aging of, 5
anatomy of, 7
back of the, examination
of, 42–43
dominant, 106

front of the, examination
of, 40–41
function of, 1–3
pressure of, 37
eye care specialist for diagnosis for macular degeneration
choosing of, 32–34
general ophthalmologists,
33
optometrists, 32–33
questions to ask, 51
retinal specialists, 34
eye examination for diagnosis
for macular degeneration
Amsler grid test, 39
of back of the eye, 42–43
eye pressure testing, 37–38
of front of the eye, 40–41
fundus fluorescein angiography, 44, 47
length of, 35–36
optical coherence tomography, 45, 47–50
preparation for, 34–35
pupil dilation, 40
range of eye movement
test, 39
routine, importance of,
72–73
visual acuity testing, 36–37
visual field testing, 38–39
eye pressure testing, 37–38
eyeglass filters, 84
eyeglass-mounted magnifiers,
82
eyelids, 40

Eylea (aflibercept), 60
F
family, engaging, 93
family history as risk factors
    for macular degeneration,
    17
    fats
    bad, 76
    choosing, 76–77
    good, 76
    monounsaturated, 77, 109
    polyunsaturated, 77, 110
    saturated, 76, 111
    trans, 76
FDA, 68
fibrosis, 44
floaters, 63, 106
fluorescein dye, 37, 106
fluorescent light bulbs, 86
fovea, 2, 106
free radicals, 18, 106
friends, engaging, 93
front of the eye, examination
    of, 40–41
fruits, 75–76
function of eye, 1–3
fundus fluorescein angiogra-
    phy, 44, 47, 106
G
games, 91
gardening, 91–92
gender as risk factors for
    macular degeneration, 16
general ophthalmologists, 33
geographic atrophy, 6, 8,
    106–107
glaucoma, 37, 107

good fats, 76
H
halogen light bulbs, 86
handheld magnifiers, 81
HDL. *See* high-density lipo-
    protein (HDL)
hemorrhage, 63
high blood pressure, 18, 73,
    107
high-density lipoprotein
    (HDL), 76, 107
home monitoring for dry
    macular degeneration, 57
hypertension, 18, 73, 107
I
idiopathic, 107
implantable miniature tele-
    scope (IMT), 67, 68–70
follow-up training sessions
    after, 70
implanting, process for,
    69–70
side effects of, 70
IMT. *See* implantable minia-
    ture telescope (IMT)
indirect ophthalmoscopy, 107
indoor self-tests, 29–30
infection, 40, 63, 107
inflammation, 21, 40–42, 107
intermediate stage of macular
    degeneration, 46
intraocular lenses, 21, 107
intraocular pressure, 107
iris, 41, 107
L
lamps, 85–86
laser photocoagulation,

66–67, 107–108

LDL. *See* low-density lipoprotein (LDL)

length of eye examination, 35–36

lens, 2, 41, 108

light-sensitive cells, 46

lighting, 85–87

lipids, 43, 108

lipoprotein, low-density, 76, 108

living with macular degeneration, 79–95
family, engaging, 93
friends, engaging, 93
low-vision specialists, 79–80
low-vision support aids, 80–86
outside support, finding, 93–94
recreation, 91–92
retinal evaluations, regular, 94
social situations, adapting to, 92–93
traveling, 90–91
vision changes, strategies for dealing with, 86–89
workplace, coping in, 89–90

low-density lipoprotein (LDL), 76, 108

low vision, 80, 85, 90, 108

low-vision specialists, 69, 79–80

low-vision support aids, 80–86
address books, 86
calculators, 85
calendars, 86
check-writing aids, 86
clocks, 85
computers, 84
eyeglass filters, 84
lamps, 85–86
lighting, 85–86
magnifiers, 81–83
phones, 85
reading machines, 85
record-keeping aids, 86
voice-activated notetakers, 86
watches, 85

Lucentis (ranibizumab), 59

lutein, 56–57, 75–76, 108

M

macugen (pegaptanib sodium), 60

macula, 1, 2, 7–8, 43, 48, 108

macular atrophy, 108

macular degeneration. *See also* specific types of
advanced stage of, 46
cataract surgery as cause of, 20–21
defined, 1, 108
development process of, 4
diagnosis for, 32–53
early detection of, importance of, 30
early stages of, 45–46
intermediate stage of, 46
living with, 79–95

overview of, 1–22
progressive, reduction of
   risks for, 72–78
risk factors for, 15–20, 111
self-testing for, 27–30
stages of, 45–46
symptoms and signs of,
   23–31, 111
treatments for, 54–71
types of, 5–15
macular dystrophy, 108
macular geographic atrophy,
   8
macular hole, 108
macular pucker, 108
macular scarring, 13
macular translocation, 108
magazines, 92
magnifiers, 81–83
magnifying glasses, 81
microscope, 37, 82, 108–109
monoculars, 83
monounsaturated fats, 77, 109
movies, 92

N

National Eye Institute, 59
National Institutes of Health
   (NIH), 55–56, 59
neovascularization, choroidal,
   11, 105
nerve
   defined, 109
   optic, 8, 37, 42–43, 109
neurologic, 109
newspapers, 92
NIH. *See* National Institutes of
   Health (NIH)

normal macula, optical coherence tomography of, 48
normal retina, 3, 8
normal vision, 10
nutrition for optimal eye
   health, 75–77
   carbohydrates, choosing,
      77
   fats, choosing, 76–77
   fruits, 75–76
   vegetables, 75–76
nutritional supplements for
   dry macular degeneration,
   55–57

O

occult wet macular degeneration, 12, 109
OCT. *See* Optical coherence
   tomography (OCT)
O.D. *See* Optometric doctor
   (O.D.)
Omega-3 fatty acids, 57, 77
ophthalmologists, general, 33,
   109
ophthalmoscope, 109
ophthalmoscopy, 42, 107, 109
optic disk, 42
optic nerve, 8, 37, 42–43, 109
optical coherence tomography (OCT), 45, 47–50
   defined, 109
   of dry macular degenera-
      tion, 49
   of normal macula, 48
   of wet macular degenera-
      tion, 50
optometric doctor (O.D.),

32–33, 109
optomoetrists, 32–33, 109
organization, 88
outdoor self-tests, 29
outside support, finding, 93–94
overview of macular degeneration, 1–22
oxidation, 109–110

P

PED. *See* Pigment epithelial detachment (PED)
peripheral retina, 42–43, 110
peripheral vision, 13–14, 26, 38–39, 68, 79, 88, 110
phones, 85
photo-sensitizing dye, 66, 110
photodynamic therapy, 63–67, 110
   performing, process for, 65–66
   side effects of, 66
photoreceptors, 5, 110
pigment epithelial detachment (PED), 12–13, 110
pigment epithelium rip, 110
polypoidal choroidal vasculopathy, 110
polyunsaturated fats, 77, 110
poor nutrition as risk factors for macular degeneration, 18–19
preparation for eye examination, 34–35
pressure of eye, 37
progressive macular degeneration, reduction of risks for, 72–78
cardiovascular disease, reduction of risk of, 73–77
nutrition for optimal eye health, 75–77
routine eye examinations, importance of, 72–73
small changes, start with, 78
pupil, 69, 110
pupil dilation, 40

Q

questions to ask eye care specialist, 51

R

range of eye movement test, 39
reading machines, 85
receptor, 110–111
record-keeping aids, 86
recreation, 91–92
remodeling, 111
retina, 2, 7, 111
   diseased, 34
   normal, 3, 8
retinal detachment, 63, 111
retinal evaluations, regular, 94
retinal fibrosis, 111
retinal pigment epithelium (RPE), 2, 46, 111
retinal specialist, 33–34, 44, 65, 111
retinopathy, 34
risk factors for macular degeneration, 15–20, 111
   age as, 16
   cardiovascular factors as,

17–18
ethnicity as, 16
existing macular degeneration as, 20
family history as, 17
gender as, 16
poor nutrition as, 18–19
smoking as, 17
sunlight exposure as,
19–20
routine eye examinations,
importance of, 72–73
RPE. *See* retinal pigment epithelium (RPE)

S
saturated fats, 76, 111
sclera, 3
self-testing for macular degeneration, 27–30
Amsler grid, 27–29
indoor self-tests, 29–30
outdoor self-tests, 29
senses, sharpening other, 89
severe wet macular degeneration, 9
side vision, practicing, 88–89
slit lamp, 37, 111
small changes, start with, 78
smoking, 17, 74
Snellen eye chart, 36, 111
social situations, adapting to,
92–93
stages of macular degeneration, 45–46
stand magnifiers, 81–82
stem cell, 111
subretinal blood, 43, 111

subretinal fluid, 111
sunlight exposure as risk factors for macular degeneration, 19–20
symptoms and signs of macular degeneration, 23–31,
111

T
tear film, 37, 41, 111
thermal laser therapy, 66–67,
107–108
tono-pen, 38, 112
tonometry, 37, 112
trans fats, 76
traveling, 90–91
treatments for macular degeneration, 54–71
drug injections, 58–63
end-stage macular degen-
eration, 67
implantable miniature telescope, 68–70
photodynamic therapy,
63–67
thermal laser therapy,
66–67
20/40 vision, 36
20/20 vision, 36, 112
types of macular degeneration, 5–15. *See also* specific
types of

U
ultraviolet (UV) light, 21, 112
UV. *See* ultraviolet (UV) light
V
vascular endothelial growth
factor (VEGF), 58, 112

vegetables, 75–76
VEGF. *See* vascular endothelial growth factor (VEGF)
VEGF-Trap, 60
video magnifiers, 83
vision
central, 10, 104
changes in, strategies for dealing with, 86–89
consistent routines, 88
contrast, increased, 87–88
lighting, improved, 87
low, 80, 85, 90, 108
normal, 10
organization, 88
peripheral, 13–14, 26, 38–39, 68, 79, 88, 110
senses, sharpening other, 89
side vision, practicing, 88–89
20/40, 36
20/20, 36, 112
visual acuity testing, 36–37, 112
visual field testing, 38–39, 112
Visudyne (verteporfin), 64
vitamin C, 56
vitamin E, 56
vitamins for dry macular degeneration, 55–57
vitreous, 13, 112
vitreous gel, 42
vitreous hallucinations, 14–15
vitreous hemorrhage, 13–14, 112
voice-activated notetakers, 86

W
watches, 85
wet macular degeneration, 6–15
classic, 11, 105
combination of classic and occult, 12
defined, 6–7, 112
development of, 4
disciform scarring in, 9, 13
early symptoms of, 25–26
macular scarring in, 13
managing, 57–58
occult, 12, 109
optical coherence tomography of, 50
progression of, 26–27
retinal pigment epithelial detachment in, 12–13
severe, 9
signs of, 43–44
vitreous hallucinations in, 14–15
vitreous hemorrhage in, 13–14
workplace, coping in, 89–90
Z
Zeaxanthin, 75–76, 112
zinc, 56, 112

About the Authors

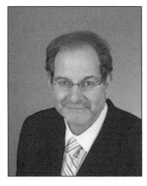 **David S. Boyer, M.D.**, is a world-renowned clinician, surgeon, and educator. He is the medical director of Retina-Vitreous Associates Medical Group in southern California. Dr. Boyer currently is a leading investigator for various national clinical trials on retinal diseases and serves as an advisor for numerous research, educational, and charitable institutions.

Dr. Boyer received his bachelor of science degree from the University of Illinois at Champaign, after which he completed his medical degree at the Chicago Medical School. In 1976, he finished his residency at the USC County Medical Center in Los Angeles. He completed his training with a yearlong retinal surgery fellowship at Wills Eye Hospital in Philadelphia.

Dr. Boyer has been a contributing author to many pivotal publications describing new treatments for retinal diseases.

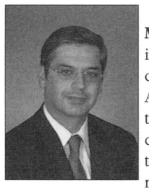

Homayoun Tabandeh, M.D., M.S., F.R.C.P., F.R.C.Ophth., is an internationally recognized retinal specialist, in practice with Retina-Vitreous Associates Medical Group. He has authored more than 150 papers, book chapters, and abstracts and has extensive experience in the field of retinal disorders.

Dr. Tabandeh trained at three world-renowned eye institutes. He completed his residency in ophthalmology at the Wilmer Eye Institute, The Johns Hopkins Hospital, in Baltimore and spent three years in retinal fellowships at the Bascom Palmer Eye Institute in Miami and Moorfields Eye Hospital in London.

Dr. Tabandeh has been an investigator in many national and international clinical trials for the treatment of retinal diseases and has received awards in research, education, and patient care. Dr. Tabandeh previously served as the director of the Retina Service, Department of Ophthalmology, University of Florida, in Gainesville.

For more information, visit: laretina.com

Consumer Health Titles from Addicus Books
Visit our online catalog at www.AddicusBooks.com

Bariatric Plastic Surgery $24.95
Body Contouring Surgery after Weight Loss $24.95
Cancers of the Mouth and Throat $19.95
Cataract Surgery $19.95
Colon & Rectal Cancer $19.95
Coronary Heart Disease $15.95
Countdown to Baby $19.95
The Courtin Concept—Six Keys to Great Skin at Any Age $19.95
The Diabetes Handbook—Living with Type II Diabetes $19.95
Elder Care Made Easier $16.95
Exercising through Your Pregnancy $21.95
Facial Feminization Surgery $49.95
LASIK—A Guide to Laser Vision Correction $19.95
Living with P.C.O.S.—Polycystic Ovarian Syndrome, 2nd Edition $19.95
Look Out Cancer, Here I Come $19.95
Lung Cancer—A Guide to Treatment & Diagnosis, 2nd Edition $14.95
Macular Degeneration—From Diagnosis to Treatment $19.95
The New Fibromyalgia Remedy $19.95
The Non-Surgical Facelift Book $19.95
Overcoming Infertility $19.95
Overcoming Metabolic Syndrome $19.95
Overcoming Postpartum Depression and Anxiety $14.95
Overcoming Prescription Drug Addiction, 3rd Edition $19.95
Overcoming Urinary Incontinence $19.95
A Patient's Guide to Dental Implants $14.95
Prostate Cancer—A Patient's Guide to Treatment $19.95
Sex & the Heart $19.95
A Simple Guide to Thyroid Disorders $19.95
Straight Talk about Breast Cancer—From Diagnosis to Recovery $19.95

The Stroke Recovery Book—A Guide for Patients and Families. $19.95
Understanding Lumpectomy—A Treatment Guide for Breast Cancer $19.95
Understanding Macular Degeneration $19.95
Understanding Parkinson's Disease, 2nd Edition $19.95
Understanding Peyronie's Disease. $16.95
Understanding Your Living Will $12.95
Your Complete Guide to Breast Augmentation & Body Contouring. $21.95
Your Complete Guide to Breast Reduction & Breast Lifts $21.95
Your Complete Guide to Facelifts $21.95
Your Complete Guide to Facial Cosmetic Surgery $19.95
Your Complete Guide to Nose Reshaping. $21.95

To Order Books:
Visit us online at: www.AddicusBooks.com
Call toll free: (800) 352-2873

For discounts on bulk purchases, call our Special Sales
Department at (402) 330-7493.
Or email us at: info@Addicus Books.com

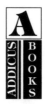

Addicus Books
P. O. Box 45327
Omaha, NE 68145

*Addicus Books is dedicated to publishing consumer health books
that comfort and educate.*